THE PUBLIC HEALTH SYSTEM IN ENGLAND

David J. Hunter, Linda Marks and Katherine E. Smith

D0280356

This edition published in Great Britain in 2010 by

The Policy Press
University of Bristol
Fourth Floor
Beacon House
Queen's Road
Bristol BS8 1QU
UK

Tel +44 (0)117 331 4054
Fax +44 (0)117 331 4093
e-mail tpp-info@bristol.ac.uk
www.policypress.co.uk

North American office:
The Policy Press
c/o International Specialized Books Services (ISBS)
920 NE 58th Avenue, Suite 300
Portland, OR 97213-3786, USA
Tel +1 503 287 3093
Fax +1 503 280 8832
e-mail info@isbs.com

British Library Cataloguing in Publication Data
A catalogue record for this book is available from the British Library.

Library of Congress Cataloging-in-Publication Data
A catalog record for this book has been requested.

ISBN 978 1 84742 462 4 paperback
ISBN 978 1 84742 463 1 hardcover

Cover design by Qube Design Associates, Bristol
Printed and bound in Great Britain by Hobbs, Southampton

Contents

List of boxes and figures

Boxes

Figures

Acknowledgements

This book grew out of a scoping study of the public health system in England commissioned by the National Institute for Health Research (NIHR) Service Delivery and Organisation (SDO) programme in 2007 to provide important background information for its new public health research initiative, which subsequently spawned seven studies. These studies will provide the material for the forthcoming books in the public health series. We are grateful to the NIHR SDO programme and to Stephen Peckham in particular, at the time academic adviser to SDO, for their support and encouragement throughout the scoping study and its transition to a book. The final report of the scoping study was greatly strengthened following comments and suggestions from several external reviewers and we are grateful for these. In addition, we received additional material from Mala Rao in personal discussion. At the time she was working in the public health group in the Department of Health leading on public health workforce issues.

The second part of the scoping study was based heavily on a series of interviews conducted with a variety of public health managers, senior executives/stakeholders across the NHS, local government and third sector. We wish to thank them for their frank and honest views, which have greatly enriched both the original study and now the book.

Finally, we wish to thank Christine Jawad, who provided invaluable administrative support to the study at various stages.

Inevitably in a book of this nature, there are many other public health advocates, researchers and practitioners who have influenced our thinking over many years. They are too numerous to list here and many have since retired or moved on. But much of our historical analysis and selection of key themes to explore has been shaped by their work and views and our interaction with many of them over the years. We should like to record our indebtedness to them as well, even though they are, for the most part, unwitting contributors.

Of course, all the views expressed in what follows remain entirely our own and are not necessarily shared by the NIHR SDO programme, Department of Health or anyone else.

List of acronyms

AHA	area health authority
ASH	Action on Smoking and Health
CAA	comprehensive area assessment
CEO	chief executive officer
CMO	Chief Medical Officer
CSCI	Commission for Social Care Inspection
DH	Department of Health
DHA	district health authority
DPH	director of public health
DsPH	directors of public health
FCTC	Framework Convention on Tobacco Control
FHSA	family health service authority
FPC	family practitioner committee
HA	health authority
HAZ	health action zone
HIA	health impact assessment
HiAP	Health in All Policies
HPA	Health Protection Agency
IA	impact assessment
IDeA	Improvement and Development Agency
IfG	Institute for Government
IOM	Institute of Medicine
JSNA	joint strategic needs assessment
LAA	local area agreement
LGA	Local Government Association
LINks	local involvement networks
LPSA	local public service agreement
LSHTM	London School of Hygiene and Tropical Medicine
LSP	local strategic partnership
MDPHF	Multi-disciplinary Public Health Forum
MoH	Ministry of Health
MOH	medical officer of health
MOsH	medical officers of health
MPH	Master of Public Health degree
NGO	non-governmental organisation
NHS	National Health Service
NICE	National Institute for Health and Clinical Excellence (formerly National Institute for Clinical Excellence)
NIHR	National Institute for Health Research

PbC	practice-based commissioning
PCG	primary care group
PCT	primary care trust
PH	public health
PSA	public service agreement
RDPH	regional director of public health
RDsPH	regional directors of public health
RIPH	Royal Institute of Public Health
RSH	Royal Society for the Promotion of Health
RSPH	Royal Society for Public Health
SDO	Service Delivery and Organisation programme
SHA	strategic health authority
SOLACE	Society of Local Authority Chief Executives
STBOP	Shifting the Balance of Power
UKPHA	UK Public Health Association
WHO	World Health Organization

About the authors

David J. Hunter is Professor of Health Policy and Management and Director of the Centre for Public Policy and Health, School of Medicine and Health at Durham University, and a Wolfson Fellow in the Wolfson Research Institute. He is also Deputy Director of the Centre for Translational Research in Public Health. His research interests include public health policy and its implementation, commissioning for health and wellbeing, and getting knowledge into practice. He has published widely in books and journals. His last book, *The health debate*, was published in 2008 by The Policy Press. He has also produced reports for organisations including The King's Fund, UKPHA, UNISON and the Local Government Association's Improvement & Development Agency. He has recently been appointed a non-executive director of NICE.

Linda Marks is Senior Research Fellow at the Centre for Public Policy and Health, School of Medicine and Health, Durham University, and a Wolfson Fellow in the Wolfson Research Institute. Her research interests include commissioning for health and wellbeing, inequalities in health, and public health policy. She has published in a range of journals, including *Public Health, Critical Public Health* and the *International Journal of Prisoner Health*, and has authored independent reports for The King's Fund, UNISON, the Health Development Agency, and others. She has previously held posts as a Fellow in Health Policy Analysis at The King's Fund and as a primary care planner in an inner London health authority, and is currently a non-executive director of Darlington Primary Care Trust.

Katherine E. Smith is a Research Fellow in Applied Policy Research in the School for Health, University of Bath. Prior to this, she worked at the Centre for Public Policy and Health, Durham University, where she spent 18 months exploring a variety of public health and social policy issues and where she undertook (with the other authors) the research on which this book is based. Katherine's research interests include health inequalities, the relationship between public health research and policy, and corporate policy influence in Europe (and its public health consequences). Recent publications include journal articles on health inequalities in a devolved Britain in *Social Science and Medicine* and *Critical Social Policy*.

ONE

Introduction

Health systems everywhere are experiencing rapid change in response to new threats to health arising from lifestyle diseases, risks of pandemic flu, long-term conditions and the global effects of climate change and other threats to sustainable development. Issues that were previously viewed as distinct and separate are now regarded as inextricably linked through their impact on health with the result that a significant refocusing of policy is under way, albeit with varying degrees of success. Such developments have profound implications for future public health policy and practice. Public health, as a function embracing a wide range of skills and expertise, is, or should be, at the forefront of this refocusing of health policy and practice. If it is to succeed, public health needs to adapt to the changing context and, in doing so, to address a number of long-standing issues that have hitherto hampered the public health function and prevented it from realising its full potential.

As the first decade of the 21st century comes to a close, this book assesses the state of the public health system in England. It is the first in a series of public health texts drawing on research largely funded by the National Institute for Health Research (NIHR) Service Delivery and Organisation (SDO) programme. The SDO launched its public health research programme in 2007, funding seven studies examining key aspects of contemporary concern and relevance to the organisation and delivery of public health. The book series will provide a platform for the findings from these studies. The purpose of this first book is to set the scene for the series by comprehensively assessing and critiquing the current state of the public health system in England. It places contemporary challenges and concerns in their historical context, tracing the dominant influence of a medical paradigm on the public health profession and exploring how this has given rise to difficulties for those who subscribe to social or structuralist paradigms. The history of public health is marked by struggles between these competing perspectives and recent policy developments have pointed in contrasting directions. While the public health profession has been actively encouraged to embrace a multidisciplinary perspective, it has simultaneously come under mounting pressure to contribute more effectively to achieving targets through clinical interventions. In the context of England, these long-standing tensions are informing ongoing debates about the purpose and nature of the public health function, how it relates to other policy sectors and its location. For many, the transfer of responsibility for most public health functions from local government to the NHS in 1974 was, and is, indicative of the fact that the profession remains an essentially narrow medical specialty that merely 'pretends' to adopt, or gives the semblance of adopting, an inclusive approach to wider concerns.

The issues outlined above form central and recurring themes throughout this book, which originated from a scoping study of public health, as the following sections explain.

On the state of the public health system: genesis of review

The genesis of the scoping study lay in the decision to provide baseline information about the development of public health policy and practice as background for the NIHR SDO's public health research programme (Hunter et al, 2007). The study was designed to be of use to the researchers submitting proposals under the call as well as to provide a stand-alone report covering the history of the public health system since 1974, focusing on significant changes in policy and structures. This is an especially active and fertile period in the evolution of public health and, while much of the earlier period has been well documented, the post-1997 era has only been partially described and analysed (Baggott, 2000; Hunter, 2003; Griffiths and Hunter (eds), 2007).

The scoping study was largely based on published literature and policy documents but, in order to gain a greater insight into how contemporary changes were being perceived, this information was supplemented by a series of semi-structured interviews with key informants. The interviewees were selected on the basis of their role in shaping public health policy and practice at the time that the interviews were conducted (in late 2006).[1] This book draws on both sources, extending and adapting the original report to take account of recent developments.

An immediate dilemma in reviewing the 'public health system' involves agreeing a definition of public health and a related set of boundaries around the notion of such a system. Public health is notoriously difficult to define with any precision because its boundaries are amoeba-like in their fluid and ever-shifting nature. It is also influenced by changing perceptions of the numerous and varying factors that impact on and shape health. Indeed, there is a great deal of overlap between the 'public health system' and broader societal, environmental, political and economic activity. The following sections discuss debates about the definitions of public health and a public health system in greater detail and help explain our own use of these terms.

A systems approach

In order to avoid an overly restrictive and reductionist account of public health and the risk of underemphasising the full extent and complexity of the public health policy arena, we decided to adopt an organising framework that would afford maximum flexibility and permit an inclusive approach. We therefore opted for a systems perspective and subscribed to the US Institute of Medicine's (IOM's) conceptualisation of a public health system as "a complex network of individuals and organizations that have the potential to play critical roles in creating the conditions for health" (Institute of Medicine, 2003: 28). As the IOM report goes on to say, these individuals and organisations "can act for health individually, but when they work together toward a health goal, they act as a system – a public health system".

Adoption of the term 'system' to describe what in reality is often a chaotic, sprawling, dynamic set of practices, which are often intensely political, and a set of activities that might more closely resemble a non-system might seem odd and is certainly open to debate. Moreover, use of the term 'public health system' risks ignoring the contribution to the public's health of anything perceived to lie outside this system, however inclusive and wide-ranging it purports to be. While mindful of this danger, we are also aware that terms like 'public health' are in common use and come with a number of assumptions and organisational arrangements in tow. Although there are few areas of policy that are devoid of influence on health, to include all of them under the rubric of a public health system would simply serve to redefine the whole of the political and economic system as a public health system. This is clearly impractical and not very helpful. In using the term 'public health system', therefore, we have sought to embrace both those organisations formally charged with taking forward the public health policy and delivery agenda, notably the NHS, local government (where the term 'wellbeing' is often used in preference to public health), and regional agencies, and also the non-governmental agencies and interest groups engaged in lobbying and campaigning in respect of various public health causes and issues such as child poverty, smoking, alcohol misuse and the provision of contraceptive services. They have had a significant impact on health policy and more generally on public policies that influence health.

Thinking about public health as a system helps demonstrate the complexity, and interrelated nature, of the issues involved (Chapman, 2004). Furthermore, it helps avoid a reductionist approach that oversimplifies reality by deconstructing problems into their component parts. The latter approach can be particularly misleading if the essential features of a problem or entity lie not in their component parts but in the interaction between them. In other words, the very act of unbundling complex issues or entities risks overlooking the interconnectedness of the issues involved, even when it is these relationships that potentially offer the most critical insights (Byrne, 1998).

Systems thinking seeks to overcome this limitation by adopting a holistic approach and analysing matters at a higher level of abstraction. It deliberately avoids focusing on the component parts (such as departments, units, individuals) and instead endeavours to maintain a focus on all underlying components in order to examine the links and interactions between them. This approach inevitably involves some loss of detail in terms of vertically drilling down through each component. However, this deficit is offset by the greater insights this approach provides in terms of understanding horizontal linkages across organisations. In characterising what is important about systems thinking, Chapman (2004) draws a distinction between 'difficulties' and 'messes'. A 'difficulty', such as fixing a car, is characterised by broad agreement on the nature of the problem and by some understanding of what a solution would involve, and there are boundaries around the time and resources required to complete the job. In contrast, a 'mess' enjoys no such certainties. Examples of 'messes' might include devising policies to cut crime, reduce obesity, or tackle binge drinking. In other words, a great many contemporary public health concerns may be considered 'messes', in Chapman's sense of the term, because there is no consensus about where the causes of the problem lie or where improvements can best be made, resulting in high levels of uncertainty. Of course, even 'messes' like public health may include particular difficulties that can be addressed through reductionist approaches. Indeed, much secondary prevention work in health may fall into this category, as there is usually a relatively high level of certainty about both the problem and its solution. However, the more the problem moves away from individuals to whole populations and communities, and from specific diseases to broader patterns of unequal mortality and morbidity, the greater the 'mess' and the less useful a reductionist approach to tackling it. For this reason, it is not a case of systems thinking and reductionist thinking competing with each other. The two are complementary and most public policy problems combine elements of both. Therefore, while we favour a public health systems approach in much of what follows precisely because it enables a holistic approach to be adopted in respect of public health challenges, we also recognise the importance of more specific and bounded contributions to understanding public health in England.

Perhaps as a consequence of the intrinsic 'messiness' of public health, the public health system can be thought of as a 'complex adaptive system', which is defined as "a collection of individual agents with freedom to act in ways that are not always totally predictable, and whose actions are interconnected so that one agent's actions changes [sic] the context for other agents" (Plsek and Greenhalgh, 2001: 626). Complex adaptive systems invariably have fuzzy boundaries, with changing membership and members who simultaneously belong to several other systems, or sub-systems. In such contexts, tension, paradox and ambiguity are natural phenomena and cannot necessarily or always be resolved or avoided. More often than not, they need to be acknowledged and managed.

We discuss the nature of the public health system in greater detail in Chapter Two but, suffice to say, we are interpreting it flexibly, acknowledging that its precise components will change over time and depending on the particular issues being focused on.

Public health function

Compounding the difficulty of adequately defining the public health system in England (and probably also elsewhere in the UK), the public health community here has long lacked a clear conception of its core purpose and raison d'être. Lewis (1986) has suggested that, for the first three quarters of the 20th century, public health was characterised by its failure to define a clear and united identity, a trend that Wills and Woodhead (2004) claim has continued into the 21st century. Lewis's account of the development of the public health profession since the end of World War I suggests ongoing tension between the widespread and multidisciplinary nature of the aims of public health, on the one hand, and the desire to develop a recognisable public health specialist discipline within medicine on the other. Not only has this tension resulted in an ever-changing terminology to describe the public health function, it has also led to inconclusive debates about the preferred location for public health specialists and the nature of the role of the public health workforce. Since 1974, intense argument has continued over how public health should be defined: whether it is a medical specialty, whether because of the wider determinants of health it is multidisciplinary and multi-sectoral, or whether it is just a specialty to which many disciplines contribute. There have also been ongoing debates about where the public health workforce, whoever that may include, is or should be located. Difficulties in defining or conceptualising the 'public health workforce', when considering all of the factors that could potentially influence health, are closely linked with the various definitions of public health reviewed in Chapter Two and with the three domains articulated by the Faculty of Public Health (2007): health protection, health improvement and health service quality improvement (see further below). It is perhaps unsurprising, therefore, that there have been significant changes and developments around the notion of the public health workforce in England since 1974 and that these have invariably reflected the shifting policy emphases on individual versus collective approaches to public health.

As a former President of the Association of Directors of Public Health, Peter Donnelly, told the House of Commons Health Committee at the time of its 2001 inquiry into public health:

> One of the difficulties of the term 'public health' is that it means different things to different people ... Public health can span everything ... The difficulty with that is that when something like public health becomes everybody's business, what is distinctive about those people who claim to practice public health and what is the added value that they actually bring to that? (House of Commons Health Committee, 2001a: xiii)

There are also tensions between a public health function that focuses on prevention and one that is involved in planning and managing health provision for existing health problems (Berridge, 2000). Responding to this gap in defining its core purpose, in 2003, the Faculty of Public Health outlined the various components of the wide-ranging public health function, grouping them into the following three domains (Griffiths et al, 2005):

- **Health improvement**: promoting healthy lifestyles and healthy environments and encompassing issues of inequality and the wider social determinants of health.
- **Health protection**: protecting people from specific threats to their health, including such activities as immunisation and vaccination, screening, injury prevention, control of infectious diseases and emergency planning.

- **Health service improvement**: bringing an evidence-based population perspective to planning, commissioning and evaluating services and interventions to ensure they are effective, high quality, safe and accessible; supporting clinical governance.

The three domains are not discrete entities but overlap and are interdependent. Each entails a sizeable remit and involves a varied mix of skills and expertise. For instance, health promotion, if done properly, demands an exceptional range of competencies as well as cross-government policy and joined-up management at several levels, an ability to work in partnership with a diverse range of agencies and professionals (each displaying particular cultural attributes and possessing its own values), and the skills to support and strengthen community action. Both the other domains are equally complex and a great deal of coordination is therefore required in those situations where all three domains are involved. This is the case for many contemporary public health issues such as, for example, teenage pregnancy or alcohol misuse where each domain can assist both in framing the actions required and in identifying the actors who need to be engaged in constructing and delivering them.

Notwithstanding wide adoption of the Faculty's three domains, there are other typologies describing the public health function. Notable among these is Holman's (1992) typology of public health movements:

- health protection
- preventive medicine
- health education
- healthy public policy
- community empowerment.

Although there is considerable overlap between the Faculty's three domains and Holman's typology, the latter is more specific about the focus of health services in the context of public health (that is, on preventive medicine). It also usefully expands the health improvement domain by specifying the incorporation of health education, wider public policy and community empowerment.

From the perspective of the Faculty's three domains, the NHS takes the lead role for all of them although it is acknowledged that the NHS cannot act in isolation and requires support from other agencies. For each of the three domains, but particularly the first two, securing public health objectives requires partnership working across the NHS, local government, the 'third sector', and businesses at both national and local levels. Holman's (1992) typology more clearly emphasises the two areas of public health activity in which the NHS is far less able to act in isolation, namely, healthy public policy and community empowerment.

The public health professionals most frequently charged with coordinating the diverse aspects of public health at a local level are directors of public health (DsPH). DsPH are accorded a key role in each of the Faculty's three domains of activity and, as a marker of the wide-ranging nature of this role, these posts are increasingly being appointed jointly between the NHS and local government. While joint posts are generally deemed to be a positive development, they nevertheless give rise to a number of concerns in relation to their accountability and precise role (Hunter (ed), 2008). Moreover, because the public health function is so complex and wide-ranging, concerns have been expressed about the potential for 'job stretch' resulting in a loss of focus and clarity of purpose. For example, such a finding was reported in an unpublished study about approaches to tackling health inequalities in Greater Manchester undertaken by the Audit Commission in 2007–08. The work was described in a presentation to the Healthcare Commission's Public Health Expert Reference Group in December 2008. Some of the same ground is covered in Fotaki's (2007) study of DsPH.

Before moving on to consider the public health workforce, this is an opportune place to make a distinction between the public health function, on the one hand, and the professional workforce, on the other, since the two do not exactly mirror each other. Indeed, it is precisely this non-alignment that often creates problems for those attempting to tackle public health concerns.

Public health workforce

As has been noted, the public health workforce is both large and diverse. In his review of the public health function and how it could be strengthened, the Chief Medical Officer (CMO) for England noted that the function is a corporate one, reflecting "the breadth of factors impacting on health and wellbeing" (Department of Health, 2001c: p 6, para 2.7). The review singled out the role of chairs, leaders and members in the NHS and local government, together with chief executives, directors of public health and others working at director level.

The report identified three broad categories as comprising the public health workforce:

- A general category embracing all those who have a role in health improvement and reducing inequalities, even where they do not recognise having such a role. This group comprises teachers, social workers, transport engineers, housing officers, town planners and so on.
- A smaller category of professionals who spend all or a major part of their time in public health practice working with groups and communities as well as with individuals. It includes health visitors, environmental health officers and community development workers.
- Finally, there are the public health consultants and specialists working at a strategic or senior management level and employed by the NHS. Specialists no longer need to come from a medical background but, if they do not, they are required to acquire the appropriate specialist expertise to enable them to practise at a level comparable with consultants in public health medicine.

Simply listing the groupings that comprise the public health workforce provides no insights into the varied and ongoing power struggles and turf wars that have been a feature of the public health function since at least the mid-1970s and that have often rendered it less effective than it might otherwise have been. Nor do the groupings convey any sense of the professional and sectoral barriers that frequently serve to disable effective and coordinated public health activity. At a macro level, for example, there is a much talked-about barrier between the NHS and local government. Within this, there are also numerous barriers between different sectors inside each of these organisations. Primary care, for example, has often been accused of failing adequately to understand or value public health and Taylor et al (1998) have identified a number of reasons for this:

- the lack of a 'shared' language – that is, shared definitions of public health between primary care practitioners and other stakeholders, including members of the community;
- poor understanding of collaborative working, both within primary health care teams and between GPs and other agencies;
- the dominance of a medical model of primary care, with its emphasis on general practice and medically dominated organisation and values;
- poor understanding of the key principles of public health among primary care professionals.

In their work with primary care organisations, Meads et al (1999) also identified a number of organisational barriers facing public health. In particular, they claim there was a lack of a public health perspective in many primary care organisations and a consequential absence of public health skills and organisational capacity to work in partnerships with local authorities and others.

While many regret such a state of affairs and insist that the NHS can be encouraged to take a more proactive approach to public health, others believe that the NHS's core business is, and always will be, to treat sickness and ill health and that, as a consequence, responsibility for focusing on health in a broader, holistic sense (that is, 'wellbeing') should lie elsewhere (Elson, 2004). Elson (2004) does not view such thinking as an attack on the 'existence or competence' of the NHS. After all, there is strong public support for safe and effective treatment services and, hence, the medical dominance within the NHS is not surprising. However, as Elson also notes, to attempt to give equal weight to the public health agenda within a service dominated by concerns with ill health presents real difficulties. This tension is echoed by the CMO for England in a forthright critique of the continuing fixation on hospital beds despite the government's "major and unprecedented commitment to public health" (Department of Health, 2006). He went on to suggest that:

> This situation has not been created by any person or group of people. It is the result of many disparate factors, but at its heart is a set of attitudes that emphasises short-term thinking, holds too dear the idea of the hospital bed and regards the prevention of premature death, disease and disability as an option not a duty. It is time for things to change. (Department of Health, 2006: 44)

In Elson's opinion, what is required is a reawakening of a sense of local government's responsibility for making "the promotion of the public's health a mainstream part of public policy once more" (Elson, 2004: 44). The use of the term 'reawakening' is intended to recall the era before the NHS when local government was far more active in public health. With the arrival of the NHS, local government gave up its traditional responsibilities for this area of public service, a development compounded by the transfer of formal public health responsibilities from local government to the NHS in 1974. From then on, anything to do with health was regarded as 'an NHS responsibility'.

While efforts have been made to conceptualise the public health workforce and equip it with the requisite skills, this task has been made more difficult and has taken longer to complete because of the high degree of turbulence and uncertainty to which the function has been subjected, especially from 1974 onwards. Although the successive waves of policy change since the 1970s have not all been directed primarily at the public health community, they have nevertheless had a major impact on policy and practice at all levels of the system. This is particularly true of those sections of the workforce employed by, or working directly with, the NHS. Successive reorganisations of the NHS since 1974, and especially over the past decade or so, have left their mark on public health. Resources and structures have often been in a state of flux, making it difficult to establish effective partnerships between organisations and individuals. A recent review of progress in meeting public health objectives since 1997 concluded that structural and other changes in resourcing "actually slowed progress in improving health and tackling inequalities in health" (Healthcare Commission and Audit Commission, 2008: 74). The review noted that "partnerships were sometimes destabilised" and "critical functions such as health promotion were lost in reorganisations and the redesign of local healthcare organisations". Frequent raids on public health budgets to support other aspects of NHS activity, especially notable in the financial year 2005–06, also hampered the delivery of local health improvement programmes. Indeed, this practice was singled out for special mention by the CMO in his 2005 annual report (Department of Health, 2006), and by Wanless and colleagues in their review of public health for The King's Fund (Wanless et al, 2007). Both were highly critical of this practice, condemning those involved for failing to focus on the long-term interests of the public's health. Several years of significant new funding for the NHS have resulted in resources being available for promoting health. However, given that the outlook for public expenditure from 2011 onwards looks grim, there is every chance such practices may recur. Public services, including the NHS and local government, will face serious cuts in funding and it remains to be seen whether those charged with making these decisions will go for easy targets, including public health programmes, as has happened in the past or adopt a more imaginative approach to managing demand by preserving investment in such initiatives and providing robust business cases for investing in them. If the new emphasis on commissioning is to carry any real substance, then a test will be the extent to which public health is accorded enough of a priority to confront rising demand and thereby ease the pressure on acute health services.

At the same time, the policy context in which public health practitioners are required to operate has shifted in recent years from one where there was an expectation that government was responsible for developing and leading collective responses to public health problems to one where far more emphasis is placed on what individuals can (and should) do for themselves, with government and other sectors, notably business, merely playing an 'enabling' role (Hunter, 2005; Dowler and Spencer, 2007). Taken together, developments over the past 35 years or so have resulted in a public health community that is increasingly insecure and unsure of its purpose, or of its fitness for whatever that purpose proves to be.

Given the diverse nature of the public health workforce, and in order to provide some agreed coherence to the skills required to discharge their functions effectively, the Public Health Skills and Career Framework was launched in early 2008 (Public Health Resource Unit and Skills for Health, 2008). This framework is designed to provide a tool for anyone, at any stage of their career, whose work involves improving people's health and wellbeing or who wishes to develop their skills and/or a career in public health, including those for whom public health is not their main area of work. The framework is intended to respond to criticisms that skills and career development in public health have traditionally focused on public health specialists, neglecting the diverse but significant contributions of others, both within and beyond the NHS. The underpinning aim of the framework was to provide a coherent and consistent vision for the public health sector. The fact that the framework was endorsed by the government in England and the devolved administrations elsewhere in the UK demonstrates its appeal.

Shifting the paradigm

Many of the concerns described above in relation to barriers to achieving effective public health, and the play of power that underpins many of them, go to the heart of debates about what the NHS is for and whether it should continue to be accorded the lead role for much of the public health function. These long-running and deeply felt concerns form the basis of a power struggle that runs throughout the history of public health in the UK and remains alive in some quarters.

Whether intentional or not there is a view that, in England and elsewhere in the UK, public health medicine has effectively hijacked broader health promotion initiatives such as the Ottawa Charter (WHO, 1986) and 'Health for All' (WHO, 1981). Those occupying health promotion or community development roles might wish to contest a presentation of public health as being dominated by values aligned to medical rather than social or structuralist paradigms. While there is a recognition that public health needs to move away from its medical roots and embrace a more multidisciplinary base, the traditional stakeholders in public health have proved adept at co-opting, or absorbing, broader public health initiatives, including those that may pose a threat to their position and authority (Lewis, 1986). Hence, many commentators remain critical of the control maintained by public health medical practitioners and the associated dominance of an agenda focusing on disease prevention and other clinically oriented targets (Hunter, 2003).

Central to the notion of a public health system is the intention of 'creating the conditions for health'. This may be directly contrasted with public health medicine's traditional focus on illness and disease, which concentrates on deficits rather than assets. As a result of the dominance of public health medicine, policy and practice has tended to adopt a deficit model (Morgan and Ziglio, 2007), focusing on the failure of individuals and local communities to avoid disease rather than developing and supporting their potential to create and sustain health. Deficit models are helpful in addressing some key public health issues but they also pose dangers, encouraging policy makers and practitioners to focus on responding to health problems that have already manifested themselves, rather than on maintaining health and preventing the occurrence of ill health.

Plan of book

The issues and themes touched on above are revisited at greater length in subsequent chapters. The purpose in introducing them here is to demonstrate how complex and contested the public health function has become. These complexities are reflected in a wide range of regional and local partnerships, which span health services, local authorities, business and the third sector. Although partnerships are clearly an important feature of the public health system, in most such arrangements there currently remain unresolved questions of remit, governance, accountability and impact, which all too often undermine their effectiveness. Engagement is increasingly viewed as key to an effective public health system as, indeed, it is to leadership more generally (Alimo-Metcalfe, 2008). This refers not only to people engaging with their own health or with a wider public health agenda but also to the ways in which a public health workforce, however defined, needs to engage with the relevant population as well as a range of other stakeholders.

These issues and themes prompt a set of fundamental questions about the role of the public health function in England, including the following:

• Is it about promoting health or allaying ill health?
• Is it about 'downstream' secondary prevention or 'upstream' primary prevention?
• Is it about influencing the collective efforts of society, led by government, or is it about helping individuals decide what is best for their health, with governments merely enabling them to make better-informed decisions through information and advice?
• If its medical roots are no longer regarded as central, then why do those with a medical background continue to hold such sway over policy and practice and over workforce issues?
• Do public health practitioners possess the requisite skills to meet the challenges that public health poses?

There are no simple answers to any of the above questions. Indeed, their very existence and persistence helps account for the puzzling paradox that, at a time when the health of the public has arguably never been higher on the policy agenda, achievements have been remarkably limited (Hunter, 2003; Wanless, 2004). These questions also help explain why there are ongoing and repeated criticisms of the function and workforce in terms of a seeming inability to manage change, work effectively in complex partnerships and secure better health outcomes. In short, these issues underpin explanations for why the current public health system remains so apparently dysfunctional and is failing to operate as an effective system.

The remainder of the book does not promise to provide comprehensive or conclusive answers to all of these long-standing, fundamental questions but it does explore the underlying issues in some detail, attempting to progress the dialogue about the public health function in England and about how it may be optimally discharged. Following this introductory chapter, the book is divided into five further chapters.

Chapter Two considers in more detail definitions of public health and how these in turn influence conceptions of a public health system. It does so in the light of the varying, and often contested, views and assumptions as to what public health is, what its guiding values are and who actually does public health. The latter is connected to consideration of the debates surrounding what is an increasingly diverse and complex workforce employed by, and working in, a variety of organisations and institutional arrangements.

Chapter Three charts in some detail the evolution of the public health system in England from 1974 to 1997, noting key features and policy developments. The cut-off year of 1997 has been chosen because the arrival of a new Labour government in May of that year marked something of a watershed for public health policy. The chapter presents an analysis of key shifts in the way that public health was understood, including the emergence of the 'new' public health in the 1970s and 1980s, following a series of international initiatives emanating from the World Health Organization (WHO), notably the Alma Ata Declaration, Ottawa Charter and *Health for all* strategy. As if to demonstrate how slow progress has been and how much remains to be done, many of the preoccupations promoted in these initiatives resurfaced decades later in the 2008 report of the WHO Commission on Social Determinants of Health (WHO, 2008a). The chapter assesses the dominance of public health medicine for much of this period and the challenges it faced from those who subscribed to political and ecological models of public health. These various perspectives underlay moves within this period to establish a multidisciplinary workforce embracing the breadth and range of public health concerns.

Chapter Four reviews the policy and organisational changes that have occurred since 1997 following the change of government. New Labour sought to accord a high priority to the health of the public and was strongly committed to putting both health improvement and health inequalities back on the policy agenda. An important symbol of this new policy emphasis was the appointment of the UK's first ever Minister for Public Health. The chapter presents and assesses the various policy developments from 1997 to the present day, including the two public health White Papers of 1999 and 2004 respectively (Secretary of State for Health, 1999, 2004). It also examines other developments affecting public health within this period, including changes in the structure of the NHS, the relaunching of commissioning under the heading 'world class commissioning', and the policy shifts towards markets and choice in the provision of health and health care.

Chapter Five is structured around a series of issues that have currently come to the fore in the public health system, all of which have their roots in the history of public health charted in the preceding chapters. These issues represent the key policy and practice challenges facing the public health system as it moves through the 21st century.

Several of the issues picked up in this chapter will form the subject of other books in the series.

Chapter Six looks ahead to some of the key threats to the health of the public and the challenges facing a public health system in future. These include climate change and environmental concerns; the need for a concern for health and wellbeing to permeate a far wider range of policies, tasks and activities than at present and become a priority for those working in fields that would not normally be considered relevant to public health; and the thorny and persistent subject of health inequalities, which, arguably, is more a matter of social justice than health policy. A strong and confident public health system will contribute effectively to meeting these challenges. The global economic crisis could also provide an opportunity to find new ways of making progress that do not compromise sustainability.

Note

[1] A total of 28 interviews were conducted between May and July 2007 (the majority – 26 – were conducted by telephone but two, at the request of the interviewees, were conducted face to face). In order to allow interviewees to speak as freely as possible, and in line with good ethical practice, individuals have not been identified and are referred to in terms of their professional location. However, it is important to underline that the interviews were specifically designed to solicit respondents' personal reflections and views, and interviewees were specifically encouraged to draw on their own experiences. Consequently, interviewees should not be perceived to be speaking on behalf of the organisations where they were employed. Overall, interviewees came from the following professional locations: four were based in the Department of Health; nine were based in strategic health authorities or regional government offices; six were based in primary care trusts; three were based in local authorities; five were based in non-governmental organisations; and one was based in a relevant professional body. The majority of potential interviewees were selected on the basis of the research team's networks and knowledge of the field, but further interviewees were suggested to the researchers as the interviews progressed and several of these were subsequently followed up. The aim was to ensure that the sample of interviewees reasonably reflected a cross-section of the public health system's component parts. Further details of the interviewing approach and process are available elsewhere (Hunter et al, 2007).

TWO

Public health and a public health system

As already noted in Chapter One, public health is a contested term, without a single or a simple definition. Its amoeba-like nature means its parameters change in line with perceptions of the key influences on the health and wellbeing of populations, while the components of a 'public health system' not only reflect how public health is defined but also inform the myriad of organisational routes through which public health problems are galvanised and addressed.

In 1948, the World Health Organization (WHO) defined health as "a state of complete physical, mental and social well-being and not merely the absence of disease or infirmity". This influential and aspirational definition appeared in the Preamble to the WHO's Constitution as adopted by the International Conference held in New York between 19 and 22 June 1946. It was signed on 22 July 1946 by the representatives of 61 States (WHO, 1948). The definition indicates the potential range of factors that can have an impact on individual health and wellbeing. By implication, it also indicates the breadth of the public health agenda, reflecting its potentially all-encompassing nature. Population health, including inequalities in health, are influenced by national fiscal and public policies, the distribution of wealth and the broader social and economic environment across the whole of the life course. Many issues with potentially devastating impacts on population health, such as climate change and new pandemics of infectious diseases, require concerted political, cross-national and global action.

Public health activities give rise to political and ethical tensions, which are reflected in debates over the boundaries of 'stewardship', defined as the collective responsibility that governments assume for protecting the health of their populations (Saltman and Ferroussier-Davis, 2000). Moral and ethical questions arise over the balance to be negotiated across personal and collective responsibility, across public and private interests, and between the rights of the community vis-à-vis personal freedoms. The question of stewardship also raises issues over the primacy of health and health improvement in policy decisions taken in other sectors, which may have a bearing on health. Stewardship in this context situates public health in a wider political context and may involve trade-offs across different sectors.

At the level of discourse, different connotations of calling an issue a 'public health problem' add further complexity. Verweij and Dawson (2007) note that the use of the term 'public health' to describe a problem can denote urgency (in epidemiological terms), responsibility (implying collective action is needed), causation (that is, influenced by issues outside the control of the individual) or moral priority. In addition to this may be added the tendency by some to delimit 'public health' by the activities of public health practitioners.

All of these aspects influence the ways in which a public health system is conceptualised, the reach of public health policy, the constitution of public health partnerships, what are seen as the boundaries between individual and collective responsibility, and the ways in which the public health function is defined and carried out by public health practitioners.

Given the close links between definitions of public health and the nature of the public health system, this chapter begins by looking at definitions of public health before discussing the parameters of a public health system.

What is public health?

As discussed, definitions of public health abound, varying between times and contexts (Hamlin, 2002; Hunter, 2003). These issues are taken up in a Nuffield Council on Bioethics (2007) working group report on ethical issues in public health, which argues that, because of the "various contexts of, and approaches to, public health action, and the many factors affecting health that could be targeted, defining 'public health' is not straightforward" (Nuffield Council on Bioethics, 2007: p 5, para 1.6). Moreover, "the many factors affecting health create problems for public health professionals and policy makers, as it is often difficult to identify a single causal factor for a specific population health problem" (Nuffield Council on Bioethics, 2007: p 5, para 1.5). This leads the working group to single out two notions as being of special importance: the *preventative* nature of public health interventions on the one hand, and their achievement through *collective efforts* on the other hand. Public health is therefore underpinned by concepts of 'public good' and 'public services'.

Similar definitional concerns are evident in the literature. Some definitions of public health are normative, others are descriptive; some focus on preventive and environmental services, while others span the wide – almost limitless – range of factors that impinge on the health of populations. It is nevertheless possible to draw out some common features of all these definitions. Public health is usually thought to concern the health of populations (rather than individuals) and, as such, often makes reference to wider determinants of health and a general sense of common interest (Beaglehole et al, 2004). Furthermore, in contrast with health care services, public health is concerned with 'moving upstream', identifying health trends and risks to health over the longer term. As Szreter (2002) points out, ascertaining the state of the public's health requires organised social interventions, including the collection of census and other population-based data, supported by the necessary resources (including people) to interpret these data. Furthermore, as population health is affected by political decisions over the distribution of material resources, it is intimately linked to social change. This requires responses that are flexible enough to adapt to what is inevitably a continually changing set of circumstances.

In 1920, Winslow defined public health as "the science and art of preventing disease, prolonging life and promoting physical health and efficiency through organized community efforts". Almost 70 years later, this early definition was echoed in an official inquiry into the public health function in the UK, which described public health as: "the science and art of preventing disease, prolonging life, and promoting health through the organised efforts of society" (Acheson, 1988). This definition has enjoyed wide acclaim both in the UK and internationally. It formed the basis of Wanless's (2004) definition in his government-commissioned review of the state of public health policy and practice in England. Wanless's argument was that "the organised efforts of society" should be interpreted in their widest sense, including not only government, public and private sector organisations, and communities, "but also the aggregate efforts of individuals in respect of their and their families' health status" (Wanless, 2004: 27). Extending Acheson's original definition, he therefore proposed what he regarded as a more appropriate definition in keeping with contemporary thinking and government public policy:

> The science and art of preventing disease, prolonging life and promoting health through the organised efforts *and informed choices* of society, *organisations, public and private, communities and individuals*. (Wanless, 2004: 23; italics indicate new words)

Within the UK, attempts to define public health have often been made in the context of the public health function – that is, the organisational arrangements designed to secure population health. As one example, the Scottish Executive defined the public health function as "a robust, adequately resourced endeavour that can secure and sustain the public health, addressing health policy issues at a population level and leading a co-ordinated effort to tackle underlying causes of poor health and disease" (Scottish Executive Health Department, 1999). The historical background to defining the public health function in the context of the public health profession is further described in Chapter Three.

Disagreements about how to define public health are not confined to the UK. In the US, the Institute of Medicine (IOM) stated that:

> … public health, as a profession, as a governmental activity, as a commitment of society is neither clearly defined, adequately supported, nor fully understood (Institute of Medicine, 1988: v)

The lack of clarity about what public health encompasses was one reason that the newly elected Labour government of 1997 requested the then Chief Medical Officer (CMO) for England, Kenneth Calman, to undertake a review of the public health function. The ensuing report was published four years later by Calman's successor, Liam Donaldson (Department of Health, 2001c). It cites the Acheson review, referred to earlier, describing public health as:

> … efforts to preserve health by minimising and where possible removing injurious environmental, social and behavioural influences, but also the provision of effective and efficient services to restore the sick to health, and where this is impracticable, to reduce to a minimum suffering, disability and dependence. (Acheson, quoted in Department of Health, 2001c: 5)

The report goes on to list five key areas for achieving 'Health for All by the Year 2000', originally outlined in the Ottawa Charter for Health Promotion, which was the outcome of the first international conference on health promotion (WHO, 1986):

• building healthy public policy;
• creating supportive environments;
• strengthening community action;

- developing personal skills;
- reorienting health services.

The CMO's report claims that most definitions of public health share important elements, namely, that a wide range of factors are involved, including "social, economic, environmental, biological and service factors" and that, consequently, "a range of agencies and organisations in all sectors of society can improve health by their actions, even if indirectly" (Department of Health, 2001c: 6). Nevertheless, debates over definition have continued in the form of extensive discussions about the public health function, leading the CMO for England to complain, in his 2005 annual report, of "constant 'navel gazing' [which] has ultimately eroded the focus and consistency of purpose of the public health function" (Department of Health, 2006: 40). While this frustration is understandable, as mentioned at the outset, the problem of defining public health and the public health function is more than a linguistic conundrum – it goes to the heart of what public health as a system is intended to do and with what means. As Mallinson and colleagues put it:

> The symbolic nature of language is part of the mechanism
> people use to position themselves as an 'insider' or 'outsider'
> in a particular interest field. (Mallinson et al, 2006: 264)

The reasons for the lack of consensus lie in large part in fundamental disagreements over the respective roles of the individual versus the collective or state (Hunter, 2005; Jochelson, 2006). These tensions have re-emerged in recent policy debates about the 'nanny state', especially in relation to so-called lifestyle factors such as alcohol and tobacco use, nutrition and exercise. WHO argues that the stewardship function of government ought to be strengthened on the grounds that protection of the public's health is a fundamental responsibility of government (Travis et al, 2002), an approach echoed in the report on ethical issues in public health published by the Nuffield Council on Bioethics (2007), which was mentioned earlier in this chapter. According to the working group, and other analysts, if there are only some things that government can do to promote health then such interventions should not be rejected as paternalistic state interference but should be regarded as the actions of an enlightened government intended for the greater good. The decision to ban smoking in public places in the Republic of Ireland in 2004, which was followed by the UK (starting with Scotland in March 2006), may be viewed as an example of this type of intervention.

A broad definition of public health, embracing social and ecological approaches, was articulated in the Foresight report on obesity (Butland et al, 2007), which echoes the holistic approach to primary health care outlined in the Declaration of Alma Ata in 1978 (and recently re-emphasised by WHO (2008c) as key to reducing inequities in health outcomes). The Declaration marked a crucial move away from narrow, professionally led conceptions of primary health care towards a more participative and multi-sectoral approach. Recognised as fundamental to population health, and therefore to a public health system, the public health aspects of primary care in the UK have been only partially exploited. Revisiting Alma Ata 28 years later, Green et al (2007) conclude that, while the Declaration remains a useful framework for assessing health systems, in the English context there remains a gap between policy and practice. Furthermore, they view the introduction of the 'choice' agenda and a market model for health as potential distractions from the purpose of achieving health improvements, arguing that these developments succeed only in widening health inequalities between social groups (Green et al, 2007).

Different approaches to defining public health described in this chapter were reflected in the interviews we undertook with key stakeholders in 2006. The term 'public health' was itself perceived as problematic by many of these interviewees because of its historical associations with sanitation, a medical model of health and a specialised workforce.

> NGO (non-governmental organisation): I do think it's a problem because it's tied up with people in the public thinking either that it's disease scares and immunisation programmes or … it's like rats and drains and things like that and they don't see health and wellbeing … as being public health … 'Public health' has been commandeered by two things: it's either been very medicalised or very environmentalised, in terms of local authorities' approach. And I think, if we've got a confused title, we've got a confused message.

Moreover, several interviewees suggested that the frequent association of the term 'public health' with the public health profession meant that important levers for change were often overlooked or ignored:

SHA (strategic health authority): It's not always helpful because different people mean different things by it, and there is always the temptation of something that comes with the label 'public health' to be considered the responsibility of the Director of Public Health. And actually the people who can probably make the biggest difference are the Chief Executives and the whole of the corporate entity of either an NHS organisation or a local authority.

Likewise, the association of 'health' with health services was perceived to pose further problems for public health:

Local government: When people say, 'oh that's a health issue', what they often mean – especially in local government – is, 'that's an NHS issue'. Now, the more we continue to say, 'oh that's a health issue therefore it's outside our sphere of influence', the less we understand that health is our business. So I think part of this is about language being really important.

While alternatives to 'public health', such as 'wellbeing', were acknowledged by many of the interviewees to have broader appeal within local government, they were also perceived to suffer from some of the issues affecting interpretations of the term 'public health', not least in terms of their inherent vagueness. Hence, alternatives were constructed largely as equally open to misinterpretation and few interviewees seemed to feel the use of new terms would do much to address the underlying problems. Furthermore, some interviewees (largely, but not exclusively, those who were attached to the professional public health community) were deeply opposed to any suggestion that the term 'public health' should be replaced:

SHA: I would be terribly opposed to any attempt to alter it. The problem is not with the term 'public health' or anyone's understanding of it; the problem is with the practice of public health and changing the title won't make any difference.

The most common suggestion for getting over the difficulties associated with the varying interpretations of 'public health' was to supplement discussions with more precise terms, depending on the context. For example, there were suggestions that it might be better to refer specifically to 'health improvement', 'health inequalities' or 'health protection', as appropriate, rather than continually to search for a less vague but nevertheless all-encompassing term.

While there were different approaches to the merits of the term, there was more agreement among interviewees about the need for a common vision, which, while also difficult to define, would be underpinned by shared values. What these values ought to involve is discussed further in the next section of this chapter.

In summary, agreeing on a definition for a subject as broad as public health is inevitably problematic and may not be possible. As Garrett (2002) surmises, while there appears to be some level of consensus, at a broad theoretical level, around the nature of public health as being something that focuses on the health of the population and that is of benefit to it, there is little consensus on how to translate broad policy statements into effective action. The absence of consensus about what public health is represents an ongoing impediment to establishing what an appropriate public health system that is fit to tackle contemporary public health problems might look like. Whatever such a system might comprise and set out to achieve, it surely needs to be governed by a coherent philosophy and clear sense of purpose. In the absence of these guiding features, it remains unclear what sort of workforce is required and with which skills and competencies it needs to be equipped.

The nature of the public health system

As noted in Chapter One, the notion of a public health system can provide a useful organising device or framework to bring together all the various sectors, statutory and non-statutory, that contribute to the public's health. We have adopted an inclusive approach to this notion, taking it to embrace both those organisations formally charged with taking forward the public health policy and delivery agenda (such as the NHS, local government and regional agencies in England), as well as the non-governmental agencies engaged in lobbying and campaigning around various public health causes and issues, such as child poverty, smoking and the provision of contraceptive services. These latter actors are important because they often provide a bridge between particular population groups and public health and policy professionals. Furthermore, they have had a significant influence on health policy and on wider public policies that influence health.

A public health system can be viewed in descriptive and historical terms – that is, as a summary of the organisations and workforce formally involved in identifying and addressing population health needs, the ways in which they interact (or fail to) and how each of these components has changed over time. It can also be viewed normatively, in terms of how the elements of such a system might be configured to address factors that influence the health of the public over the short and the longer term. The key point is that any critical assessment of a public health system has to address the extent to which that system, as currently configured, is capable of identifying and addressing both present and projected public health challenges. It is in identifying these challenges, and determining the appropriate response in organisational and workforce terms, that many of the deep-seated tensions already touched on in Chapter One begin to emerge.

In this section we are concerned with the public health system in both descriptive and historical terms. (Chapter Five explores how such a system might function differently, and possibly more effectively, in the light of changes currently being implemented.)

Adopting a descriptive and historical perspective helps illustrate how locations, responsibilities and systems of accountability within the English public health system have changed over time. It also encourages us to reflect on the benefits and costs of various reorganisations on the effective operation of this system. The following section explores conceptualising the public health function as a system and considers whether it provides a means of addressing long-standing concerns around public health governance and accountability. We begin by considering the notion of a public health system as a way of encompassing the key factors that influence health and then go on to describe a number of different approaches to operationalising this broad concept, drawing on international examples as well as ones from England.

Whole systems approach

The public health system can encompass all of the factors influencing the health of populations, including proximal causes as well as wider social determinants such as social exclusion, poverty, housing and education. To the extent that definitions of health are global, encompassing and aspirational, so the landscape of the public health system expands. As mentioned earlier, the WHO concept of health as a "state of complete physical, mental and social wellbeing and not merely the absence of infirmity" leaves little outside the potential purview of public health. Consequently, this definition may be regarded as naive, unrealistic and utopian. Nevertheless, many observers consider that it provides a good starting point (Calman, 1998), usefully highlighting that health is multidimensional and holistic, embracing all aspects of individual and collective existence. A healthy person is one who enjoys a harmonious existence within themselves and within their societal and environmental contexts.

One influential reminder of the importance of adopting a whole systems approach to public health has been Dahlgren and Whitehead's 'rainbow diagram' (see Figure 2.1), which helpfully illustrates both the limitations of isolated downstream interventions and the complex ways in which social factors (and ways of addressing them) are interrelated (Dahlgren and Whitehead, 1991). It identifies the range of sectors at both national and regional levels that influence the health status of populations, the sectors across which action would need to be taken in relation to problems affecting the health of populations and the potential contribution of public health partnerships at both horizontal and vertical levels.

Figure 2.1: The main determinants of health

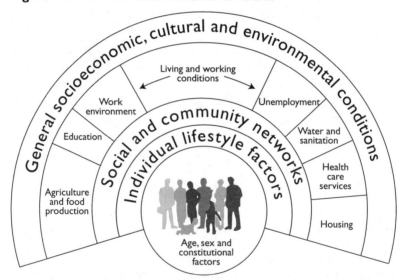

Source: Dahlgren and Whitehead (1991)

Since the diagram first appeared 18 years ago, there has been a growing awareness of health as a global issue and of the current threats to global health, including bioterrorism, climate change and potential pandemics such as the SARS and swine flu outbreaks in 2003 and 2009 respectively. There is therefore an important (and growing) global element to health protection that needs to be reflected in countries' individual public health systems. At the other end of the spectrum, there is also now a rather better understanding of some of the proximal factors that can influence wellbeing and positive health. These developments have contributed to the construction of a revised version of the 'rainbow model' (see Figure 2.2). In the final chapter, we consider the links between climate change, the environment and public health in more detail as they constitute perhaps the biggest challenge facing not just our health but our very existence.

Figure 2.2: Global determinants of health

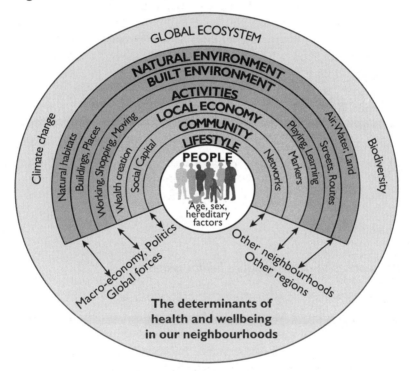

Source: Based on Dahlgren and Whitehead (1991), amended by Barton and Grant (2006) and the UK Public Health Association (UKPHA) Strategic Interest Group

The Dahlgren and Whitehead diagram, and its 2006 variant, provide a template against which the breadth and priorities of the public health system can be gauged. They demonstrate the difficulties in drawing boundaries around public health systems, illustrating the multiple levels at which action needs to take place and across which partnerships are likely to be required. They also point to the inevitable tensions between the ways that a formal public health system is constructed and the areas that lie outside it.

The idea of a public health system is not exactly novel and draws heavily on WHO's conception of a health *system* (as distinct from a health *service*), which, in turn, influenced the emergence of the 'new public health' movement, the notion of 'healthy public policy' (Milio, 1981), and the development of social and ecological models of public health, which draw on 'whole systems' and complexity thinking (Glouberman, 2000; Hunter, 2003, 2007b). These models are currently undergoing something of a resurgence, providing both an antidote to public policy interests in markets, competition and consumers, and a recognition that the public health and sustainability agendas share many of the same concerns and perhaps ought to be regarded as a single, broad agenda for action and policy change. A social, ecological and whole systems approach means working collaboratively across complex systems and with local communities and requires the development of new social indicators to match. These include measures of 'social capital' (Putnam, 2001) and psychosocial determinants of health – such as levels of social support, involvement in social networks and levels of trust and reciprocity, all of which are now understood to be closely linked to health and wellbeing (Kawachi et al, 1997; Wilkinson and Pickett, 2009). The public health system, therefore, is not just a collection of discrete entities and responsibilities. Its effectiveness is indicated by the quality of relationships across the various organisations, policies and individuals involved.

Approaches to defining public health systems

The conceptualisation of the 'public health system' put forward by the US Institute of Medicine (IOM), mentioned briefly in Chapter One, adopts a more flexible, network-based approach. The 1988 IOM report conceived of the 'public health system' as encompassing "activities undertaken within the formal structure of government and the associated efforts of private and voluntary organizations and individuals" (Institute of Medicine, 1988: 42). A second, follow-up IOM report expands the notion of a 'public health system' to describe "a complex network of individuals and organizations that have the potential to play critical roles in creating the conditions for health. They can act for health individually, but when they work together toward a health goal, they act as a system – a public health system" (Institute of Medicine, 2003: 28). While acknowledging the crucial importance of government public health agencies, the health delivery system and academic public health, this conception of the 'public health system' also specifically identifies a range of actors in wider society who play an important role in public health (see Figure 2.3).

Figure 2.3: The intersectoral public health system

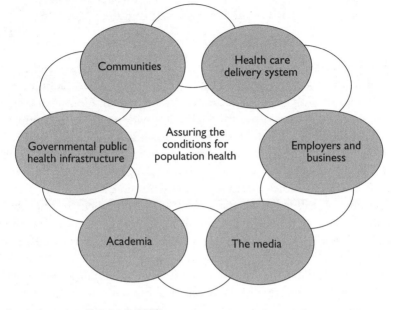

Source: Institute of Medicine (2003)

The IOM's approach is not especially novel or unique and similar conceptualisations of the public health system have been put forward in England (Ellis, 2005) as well as the rest of the UK, but what is particularly helpful about the IOM's reports is their attempt to describe the whole system in such an explicit manner. Moreover, by expanding the boundaries of the conceptualisation of the 'public health system' to agents beyond the 'usual suspects', the IOM seeks to put public health firmly on people's agendas, promoting collective rather than individual action:

> Acting alone, persons of means may procure personal medical services and many of the necessities of living. Yet no single individual or group can assure the conditions needed for health. Meaningful protection and assurance of the population's health require communal effort. The community as a whole has a stake in environmental

protection, hygiene and sanitation, clean air, uncontaminated food and water, safe blood and pharmaceutical products, and the control of infectious diseases. These collective goods, and many more, are essential conditions for health, but these 'public' goods can be secured only through organized action on behalf of the population. (Institute of Medicine, 2003: 22)

The aim of this revised conception of a 'public health system' is to expand the focus on public health to all actors whose actions are likely significantly to influence public health, which, adopting a social determinants model of health, includes a wide range of individuals and organisations:"There is strong and growing evidence that 'healthy' public policy must include consideration of domains that are not traditionally associated with health but whose influences have health consequences (eg the education, business, housing, and transportation domains)" (Institute of Medicine, 2003: 34). The focus on 'healthy' public policy outlined in the first IOM report is retained but the need to work with multiple actors to achieve the kinds of changes necessary for 'healthy' public policy to work is brought to the fore in the 'intersectoral public health system' described in the follow-up report.

Although the concept of the public health system can be applied to an almost endless range of sectors, the report's authors select five genres of actor that they feel, "together with the government public health agencies, are in a position to act powerfully for health".These are:

- 'communities', which include all the organisations and associations that make up civil society, including schools, law enforcement and so on;
- the health care delivery system;
- employers and business;
- the media;
- 'academia'.

The report goes on to outline the rationale for the involvement of each of these groups in terms of both what they can contribute to public health and what the incentives are for them to take on this role. For example, it is claimed that:"businesses and employers will have healthier workforces and constructive relationships with the community, the media will better serve the public interest, and communities will be active participants and even leaders in their own health improvement process" (Institute of Medicine, 2003: 31).

In order for the authors' concept of an effective intersectoral public health system to function, they identify the following six necessary areas of action and change:

- adopt a *population health approach* that builds on evidence of the multiple determinants of health;
- strengthen the governmental public health infrastructure – the *backbone* of any public health system;
- create a new generation of *partnerships* to build consensus on health priorities and support community and individual health actions;
- develop appropriate systems of *accountability* at all levels to ensure that population health goals are met;
- assure that action is based on *evidence* (see Box 2.1);
- acknowledge *communication* as the key to forging partnerships, assuring accountability and utilising evidence for decision making and action (Institute of Medicine, 2003: 33-4).

As this list highlights, the role of partnerships is critical to the process of achieving significant improvements in population health (see Figure 2.3 earlier in this section). Elsewhere, the report places a great deal of emphasis on community involvement and ownership in taking forward the kinds of changes it hopes to see emerge.

Box 2.1: Evidence-based policy and practice

In addition to marking an important change in central government's approach to public health (Department of Health, 1997, 1998a, 1999), the election of New Labour in May 1997 marked the start of an era in which an ethos of 'evidence-based policy' has been strongly promoted (Cabinet Office, 1999). Around the same time and specifically in relation to public health, the UK's national drive towards evidence-based policy was reinforced by international calls "to adopt an evidence-based approach to health promotion policy and practice" (WHO, 1998a). However, while the idea of basing policies on the best available evidence seems innately attractive, it is not unproblematic (Davey Smith et al, 2001; Tenbensel, 2004), particularly in the context of the kinds of 'messes' (Chapman, 2004) involved in public health, where the evidence is usually complex and contested. For many contemporary public health challenges, such as tackling health inequalities and reducing obesity, a mass of research has been undertaken and yet competing claims about both the key causes and the most promising solutions remain. Consequently, unravelling recommendations on which to *base* policy and practice decisions is far from being a straightforward task in public health.

Indeed, even in the context of evidence-based medicine, it has been argued that the complexity of evidence can mean the idea of being able to base decisions on research is fundamentally flawed (see Goldenberg, 2005).

Nevertheless, a range of initiatives has been undertaken since 1997 to try to promote the links between public health research and policy, including the creation of the Health Development Agency in 2000, which was charged with responsibility for developing the evidence base to improve health and reduce health inequalities. In 2005, this body was incorporated into the National Institute for Clinical Excellence. The new merged body, known as the National Institute for Health and Clinical Excellence, has retained the NICE acronym. To some, this move suggests a demotion in the importance of public health evidence as compared to clinical evidence, and further underlines the location of public health responsibilities within the NHS. However, NICE has sought to work hard to engage with a wide range of stakeholders, particularly those beyond the NHS, and its focus on the evidence base for multidisciplinary public health is retained by the Centre for Public Health Excellence within NICE (Kelly, 2007). There is an acknowledgement that public health interventions are complex and multifaceted, and give rise to particular issues and challenges that make them inappropriate to compare with medical or clinical interventions. The enlarged NICE is also taking forward the suggestion in Wanless's second report that studies of the cost-effectiveness of public health interventions ought to be undertaken. Indeed, it is one of the few recommendations in the Wanless report that has, so far, been acted on. Nevertheless, given that NICE responds to requests to produce guidance from the Department of Health, sets standards for good health care and is identified mainly with evidence-based medicine and clinical cost-effectiveness, there remains an issue about how far its guidance is welcomed and received by, and/or can be expected to impact on, local government, where NICE is often not recognised and has little authority.

The IOM's notion of a 'public health system', which those involved in public health have attempted to employ to ensure population health and health improvement become a driving force for action in a wide variety of sectors, has equivalents elsewhere. In Australia, for example, the New South Wales (NSW) Health Department (2001) has developed the idea of 'capacity building', which it describes as "the 'invisible work' of health promotion ... the 'behind the scenes' efforts by practitioners that increase the likelihood that effective health promotion programs will be sustained". This includes activities as diverse as exploring the opportunities for a particular programme, gathering support for relevant initiatives, developing skills of relevance to public health, supporting policy development in ways that are sympathetic to promoting health and guiding the establishment of effective partnerships. As with the IOM's notion of a 'public health system', the aim of capacity building is to increase the range of people, organisations and communities able to address health problems by establishing a common goal and purpose among a wider group of actors. This approach is similarly sympathetic to the social determinants of health model, aiming, in particular, to address health problems arising from social inequity and social exclusion.

Rather than mapping the various agents involved in the 'public health system' and the roles they might undertake, however, capacity building aims to develop sustainable skills, structures and resources for health improvement across a range of sectors. The aim is not only to secure an expanded commitment to health improvement among various communities and organisations but also to enable these agents to increase their capacity to fulfil their public health role. There is no clear prescription for how this will be achieved. Indeed, capacity building is variously referred to as "a means to an end", "an end in itself" and "a process". The NSW Health Department accepts that different organisations are likely to have quite different ways of conceptualising the notion but the model outlined suggests capacity building work exhibits several fundamental features. First, it ought to link key areas for strategy development (organisational development, workforce development, resource allocation, partnerships and leadership) to infrastructure development, programme sustainability and enhanced problem solving. Second, the Department highlights the importance of taking 'context' into account when developing capacity building strategies. Third, although capacity building activity might be developed by individuals, organisations or communities, particular emphasis is placed on the importance of developing partnerships *between* these various actors.

Whatever the theoretical models of public health systems being developed in various countries and settings, the actual policy contexts that influence the health of the public are of growing concern, especially given the increase in lifestyle-related illnesses caused by obesity, alcohol misuse and other behaviours. There is now a consensus, both in the UK and in other countries, that the challenges facing public health require multi-sector responses (Hunter, 2003). For example, in recognition of the fact that health status is largely determined by factors outside the domain of health care that instead have their roots in the ecological and social contexts in which people live, the notion of Health in All Policies (HiAP) was the main health theme of the Finnish Presidency of the European Union in the latter half of 2006 (the EU Presidency rotates on a six-monthly basis). The Finnish Minister of Health and Social Services explained HiAP in the following terms: "[It] highlights the fact that the risk factors of major diseases, or the determinants of health, are modified by measures that are often managed by other government sectors, as well as by other actors in society" (Stahl et al, 2006). HiAP can be regarded as a virtuous cycle in political and economic terms since investing in health and improving the health status of European populations (or anywhere else for that matter) "will contribute not only to increased well-being but also to economic stability and growth" (Wismar et al, 2006: xxiv). However, it should also be acknowledged, particularly in light of the current global economic recession, that a vicious cycle is also a possibility, whereby a decline in economic performance and health status puts added pressure on health care systems and health, and limits the resources available to governments to intervene.

On the other hand, there is a school of thought that maintains that economic recessions can be good for health because they may result in healthier lifestyles as a result of eating and drinking less and walking more (Ruhm, 2000). Ruhm reached his conclusions having plotted US death rates and health behaviour against economic shifts and jobless rates from 1972 to 1991, which included the recessions of 1974 and 1982. When the economy weakens, Ruhm found that people smoke less, are less likely to drink heavily and tend to exercise more. Moreover, it is the least healthily behaving people who make the biggest health behaviour changes. What might explain these findings? Given that inequalities in income between the richest and the poorest sections of society are a strong predictor of the health of populations as a whole (Wilkinson and Pickett, 2009), recessions may have a paradoxical and counterintuitive effect. Changes in consumption patterns may have a beneficial impact on lifestyle-related diseases. But the negative effects of a recession on health should not be overlooked or underestimated. The impact of unemployment on health, for example, has been clearly demonstrated although, even here, the nature of employment can have a significant impact on health outcomes. As Ruhm also found in his study of earlier recessions, mental health suffered most and, although people were possibly physically healthier, they were not necessarily happier (Ruhm, 2000).

Whatever the likely impact on health of economic downturns, what is not in doubt is the enormity of the implementation challenge that will decide HiAP's fate and ensure that health remains high on the policy and political agendas. Barriers include the departmentalism that frequently characterises government activity and renders problematic the emergence and sustainability of the cross-sectoral linkages needed to ensure effective and coordinated action (Ling, 2002). Policies to tackle a complex, cross-cutting public health issue, such as childhood obesity, can become subject to the silo-driven, vertical nature of much public policy (Hunter, 2003; Chapman, 2004). In contrast, HiAP is a horizontal, policy-related strategy and, as its advocates state in sobering terms, because the approach is part of a complex policy making process, "success should not be presumed to be easy or without complications" (Sihto et al, 2006: 17). A long-term perspective is needed, alongside a commitment to investing in appropriate research and training. The health sector also has a crucial part to play in the "vigilance of HiAP" (Ollila et al, 2006: 276). This requires having sufficient capacity in terms of public health resources at various levels to ensure that health implications are taken into account in non-health sectors. Without such a focus, the likelihood is that health sector professionals will confine their activities to curative services, or at best to disease prevention and health promotion *within* the confines of the health service sector.

Moving away from the ambitious and wide-ranging conception of the public health system underlying HiAP, the English Department of Health's website (2007a) more prosaically describes the 'modern public health system' as incorporating the following ten core functions:

- health surveillance, monitoring and analysis;
- investigation of disease outbreaks, epidemics and risks to health;
- establishing, designing and managing health promotion and disease prevention programmes;
- enabling and empowering communities to promote health and reduce inequalities;
- creating and sustaining cross-government and intersectoral partnerships to improve health and reduce inequalities;
- ensuring compliance with regulations and laws to protect and promote health;
- developing and maintaining a well-educated and trained, multidisciplinary public health workforce;
- ensuring the effective performance of NHS services to meet goals in improving health, preventing disease and reducing inequalities;
- research, development, evaluation and innovation;
- quality assuring the public health function.

While this list suggests that a public health system does indeed exist in England, despite appearances, a more detailed conceptualisation of what such a system involves is currently lacking. Each one of the elements outlined above could be described as having its own system, although degrees of complexity (and the need to link across different systems) will vary. For instance, the Foresight report on tackling obesity views obesity as a complex system involving both biological and social factors (Butland et al, 2007). What the Foresight report is particularly good at highlighting is that obesity, like many other public health concerns, is not the product of biological changes but of changes in the external environment. To capture this important distinction, the report refers to an "obesogenic environment", terminology that deliberately serves to expose and compound the "biological vulnerability of human beings". In terms of how obesity might be tackled, the report is clear that "the complexity and interrelationships of the obesity system ... make a compelling case for the futility of isolated initiatives" (Butland et al, 2007: 10). Rather, the authors argue that "a cross-cutting, comprehensive, long-term strategy" is required to bring together multiple stakeholders (Butland et al, 2007: 10). This poses a major challenge not just to medical and public health professionals but also for "governance and decision-making" more generally (Butland et al, 2007: 12). Such an approach will entail confronting vested interests in the food and drinks industry in much the same way as governments have had to confront the tobacco industry over the impact of smoking on health (Freudenberg and Galea, 2007).

Although obesity is presented as an example of a particularly complex public health issue, the Foresight report notes that obesity is not unique, having much in common with a number of other challenges to the health of the public as well as to public health practitioners. Indeed, the wider determinants of health, sometimes referred to as the 'causes of the causes', are depicted by the authors as essentially the same for most public health concerns: "The social, infrastructural and environmental factors that need to frame the planning and implementation of policies for obesity coincide with many other public health issues" (Butland et al, 2007: 13). As the report also emphasises, many of the UK's contemporary public health challenges are unlikely to be solved by exhortations for greater individual responsibility or short-term fragmented initiatives. These points are echoed in regard to the social determinants of health more generally in a recent report on the evidence base for tackling social determinants presented to the WHO's Commission on Social Determinants of Health (Kelly et al, 2007). The Commission's final report published in August 2008 (discussed in more detail in Chapter Five) reiterates these arguments (WHO, 2008a).

When combined with evidence of the failure of recent initiatives to deliver significant public health achievements, such critiques of existing policy responses and institutions suggest that current approaches to a public health system fall woefully short of the required response. While the list of elements making up England's public health system provided by the Department of Health clearly suggests that it is multidisciplinary and involves intersectoral partnerships, no detail is provided as to precisely who is involved in these arrangements and what role(s) they are expected to undertake. In an attempt to make sense of the wide range of public health related activities, the framework produced by the Faculty of Public Health (2007) to describe the public health function has been widely endorsed as a reasonable statement of what this function is about. As set out in Chapter One (see pages 6-7), this framework depicts the public health function as consisting of three overlapping domains: health protection, health improvement and health service quality improvement.

A complex system of advisory bodies, arm's length bodies and shared responsibilities populates each of these domains, further complicating matters. The National Institute for Health and Clinical Excellence (NICE) is currently developing evidence-based guidance for public health interventions, and the former Healthcare Commission monitored core and developmental standards for public health through its Annual Health Check. The Care Quality Commission, which replaced the Healthcare Commission in April 2009, has yet to decide how it intends to monitor public health, although it remains committed in principle to improving health outcomes. However, various public health functions are dispersed across multiple organisations, operating at different levels and embracing the NHS, local government and non-governmental organisations (NGOs). Health protection, for example, is regarded as a "new concept that has gained popularity as an area of public health activity in the last decade" (Nicoll, 2007: 259), which overlaps with environmental public health and is divided between the national Health Protection Agency, the NHS and local government (and is further described in the following chapter). Health improvement is similarly dispersed across a range of agencies, although with less focus around a single agency. The NHS is accorded the lead role for health improvement, although it is recognised that partnership working across the NHS and local government, including other stakeholders, is essential. There is also a major emphasis in this domain on issues around neighbourhood renewal and urban regeneration, and on area-based initiatives. Finally, health service improvement is regarded as principally an NHS function, led by the director of public health (DPH) in each organisation, although whether such a responsibility is appropriate or should comprise a core part of the public health function is not without its critics (Hunter, 2003).

While this review is concerned with all three domains and their interaction, its primary focus is on the second domain, which is where debate over the nature of the public health function and the boundaries of formal (and informal) public health systems has been most intense. Reference is made to the other domains as and where appropriate. The origins of conceiving public health in terms of these three domains "lie in the historic importance of the control of communicable disease, health education and the role of hospital and community services over the past 150 years" (Griffiths et al, 2005: 910). According to Griffiths et al (2005), conceptualising the breadth of public health within the framework of these three domains of practice is intended to make the management task more practicable. In respect of any public health problem, the domains can help both to frame the actions required and to identify those who need to be engaged in constructing public health responses. They can also be employed to understand the skill mix needed by those delivering services. However, the domains could stand accused of failing to address what has been described as the philosophical lacuna in public health in the aftermath of the Second World War when public health "allowed itself to become defined by the activities it undertook" and the idea behind it "remained indistinct" (Lewis, 1986: 3). Moreover, many leading figures in public health question whether splitting the discipline into three domains is helpful when problems may cut across these domains and require a mix of skills – for a selection of views on this point, see *ph.com* (2007). There is also a concern that the three domains remain largely NHS focused with an inevitable concentration on downstream solutions. Although this is not unimportant, it is widely agreed that these kinds of interventions will be insufficient to meet some of the most pressing contemporary public health problems, such as the challenge set out by the Foresight report in respect of obesity (Butland et al, 2007). In the light of these difficulties, it may be that, in future, topic-based specialisation will occur, with a consequent blurring of the three domains.

Defining the public health system in England, therefore, becomes quite a complex task, and one that is compounded by the absence of a coherent approach or an explicit and agreed notion of a system against which current activities can be assessed. This is reflected in key debates within public health, health promotion and general practice.

In the meantime, however, the public health infrastructure at both national and local levels remains weak and fragmented. The tensions outlined above have undermined a coherent and sustained approach, and longer-term public health priorities forever fall prey to immediate demands emanating from the health care system. These concerns were reflected in the views of the key stakeholders we interviewed when we asked them to express their views about the nature of a public health system.

Interviewees reflected the broad and inclusive definitions of the ideal public health systems discussed above and consistently emphasised that such systems should encompass far more than the limited range of organisations and individuals with 'public health' in their titles:

> PCT (primary care trust): Ideally, the public health system would include all of those elements of the socially created environment – the policies, the institutions and the means by which we govern ourselves that have an impact on health.

Moreover, reflecting the IOM approach described earlier, the importance of networking and 'joining up' was highlighted:

> PCT [different interviewee from above]: I think it is all the elements required to deliver public health programmes in a connected and joined-up way, at various levels. So, it's not just local level, it's how the system actually comprises things that are local, regional and national level as well. So interconnectedness across and also up and down.

One of the key problems that interviewees articulated in relation to the current public health system involved the current lack of connectivity between its different component parts. Their comments suggest this is evident at a variety of levels of the system, from the absence of policy coherence at central government level, to the difficulty in ensuring all the necessary parties are actively involved in public health activities at local levels:

> SHA: I would probably question the notion that there is actually a public health system. I think we have public health components of a number of different other systems and that might be part of the problem really … I think the system has developed in a rather chaotic way … and I think the pattern is very different in different parts of the country. I worked in [one region] before, and I've come to [another region] and I've found that the culture and the way of doing things, the priorities, are all completely different.

> NGO:We just have not got the right people at the table yet in terms of public health systems. And I would particularly cite people like ... planners, people who design transport systems, local government responsibility for spatial planning. I think in some areas there are bits of economic planning and economic regeneration, [which] are aware of health and the issues but they're not at the table.

It was noticeable that, when discussing the current public health system, several of the specialist health professionals – DsPH and regional directors of public health (RDsPH) – focused rather more on definitions developed by the Faculty of Public Health and public health professionals than other interviewees. For example, the Faculty of Public Health's (2007) 'three domains' of public health (see Chapter One) and the CMO's three-part definition (see Chapter Four) were both cited by interviewees who held public health professional posts. As well as contrasting with the far broader ways in which most of the interviewees described an ideal public health system, these descriptions of public health differed markedly from the descriptions provided by interviewees based in, or with strong connections to, local government. Interviewees in non-NHS posts tended to emphasise the limited nature of specialised, NHS-based public health professionals and organisations. For example:

> NGO: They [the NHS] are only small, part players in the total picture so, in my view, far more important than the NHS is getting local government on side because it's local government that will make or break the building blocks.

> Local government: I view the public health workforce as not just the NHS-employed workforce, but I think that that is not necessarily a common view of the world. I view the departments I'm in charge of to be a huge part of the public health workforce and capacity in this city, and I think it's one that isn't always, as it should be, recognised as such.

It is important, however, not to overemphasise this difference as most of the interviewees who defined the public health system in a narrow, specialist or professionalised sense were still keen to acknowledge the important role of local government and other sectors, and most of those who described the system in a broader, outcome-focused manner did also recognise the role of the specialist public health workforce.

However, there were clearly contrasting perspectives in terms of the weight that interviewees in different sectors placed on the various dimensions of public health. This suggests, as many of the interviewees explicitly stated, that, despite policy pronouncements about the broad and multidisciplinary nature of the public health workforce, work is still needed in this area.

Views on how to overcome the ongoing focus on NHS-based and medical approaches to public health varied between interviewees. Some felt a greater focus on the role of local government, in line with recent developments, would provide the required counterbalance to NHS-focused activities. However, several interviewees felt more significant organisational changes were required for England to achieve an effective public health system. As illustrated in the quotation below, suggestions were sometimes based on the idea that it was necessary to develop a new and more autonomous 'public health system', rather than merely to promote better connections across relevant agencies:

> SHA: I would like a formal fundamental review of public health systems in the country, involving all of the stakeholders, so particularly public involvement, county councils and local authorities, and probably not led by the NHS because that would give it too much of an NHS focus. And I would like to see it develop into a Department of Health based, public health structure, maybe a beefed-up Chief Medical Officer's office with a hierarchical and performance-managed structure beneath that, which had its own funding streams – so it's not subject to raiding by local NHS, or by local government executives – and a defined budget for public health and a defined series of expectations and objectives which were properly performance managed and monitored.

Relating to these tensions, interviewees also expressed some concerns about the boundaries of the 'public health system'. For example, several interviewees pointed out that broad definitions could seem to encompass almost everything, making it difficult to know how to focus public health activities and where to set limits to make the work manageable. However, at the same time, narrower definitions were perceived by most interviewees to fail to provide adequate room for public health activities addressing the wider determinants of health.

The various perspectives on the basic phrases and concepts relating to public health, including the very term itself, point to the need for some conceptual and educative work to promote shared understandings of commonly used terms and, more ambitiously, to develop the notion of a public health system. This idea was remarked on by a number of the interviewees, who felt the key to achieving desirable public health outcomes lay with an ability to instil a widespread commitment to a common vision of public health. For example:

> SHA: I think one of the key things, and it's something that we're lacking ... is a system that knows itself and a system that can describe itself, and I'm not sure that any of us in the public health community have put enough resources into the conceptual development of the system to be able to do that.

The above interviewee and several others felt that clear and widely shared goals were required and that these should be linked to a focus on outcomes rather than processes or outputs. This implies, as the following interviewee overtly describes, that an effective performance management system is required in order to facilitate and encourage clear agreements about the roles and responsibilities of the various component parts of the system:

> PCT: What I would like to develop ... is a single public health function for the city that incorporates elements of the local authority and the PCT, the NHS and the voluntary and community sector and the local NHS providers and so on so that, in five years' time, there are loads of people working in public health in the city, some of whom are employed by one organisation, some are employed by another organisation but with clear aims, clear objectives, performance managed as a coherent enterprise.

The establishment of shared goals, targets and performance management systems was seen by many of the interviewees as a key potential change that could encourage effective partnership working. The notion that working in partnership is crucial for achieving public health objectives was widely supported by interviewees and it is therefore unsurprising that many of them suggested this was an area that they would like to see policy makers tackle in the near future.

Interviewees' desire for shared goals and targets further underlines the demand for some conceptual work around the development of a public health system. The hope expressed by many of the interviewees was that, if a shared understanding of the values and dimensions of a public health system could be achieved across all relevant sectors, then public health policies and activities would benefit from a new sense of coherence, allowing public health problems to be tackled with truly multifaceted approaches. Aspirations towards the 'mainstreaming' of public health in this way contrast significantly with interviewees' accounts of the current, disjointed reality.

Unsurprisingly, in the light of interviewees' frequent comments about the varied understandings of the term 'public health', few attempted to articulate what this common vision might look like. However, there was a significant degree of consensus about the values that ought to underpin an effective public health system. The most frequently mentioned of these was a commitment to equity or fairness, which several interviewees related directly to the need to tackle health inequalities.

The second most commonly mentioned value related to the need for a public health system to be 'enabling' or 'empowering' – that is, that it should act as a system that actively engages the public and communities in health-related activities and associated decision-making tasks, rather than a paternalistic system in which public health is something that is 'done to' people. For example, some interviewees emphasised the key role that communities could potentially play in galvanising action on public health issues, when they truly believed that their input would be valued. However, at least one interviewee felt that the dominance of the medical model of public health was also a potential barrier to making effective progress on this front, as, until this way of thinking diminished, it was unlikely that genuine or sustained public engagement would be forthcoming.

The third value that interviewees emphasised was a widespread commitment to the idea that an effective public health system should help address issues relating to social justice and social exclusion – that is, that it would focus on wider social determinants of health as well as trying to change individuals' lifestyle behaviours. Several of the interviewees who focused on the need for greater policy coherence suggested that this issue was linked to the ability to create a public health system that was effectively able to grapple with wider social and economic determinants of health. If public health values could be mainstreamed, the hope, to quote the following interviewee, was that broader (non-health) policies, at the local and national level, could be 'public health proofed':

> NGO: I think there has to be a revisiting of some of those fundamental policy commitments of the past ten years, so you have to do something about child poverty. We have to do something about making it worthwhile for people to work. I think what we need to do is kind of public health proof, if you like, a lot of other policies that actually have a direct impact.

The mainstreaming of public health goals to this extent presupposes that shared public health outcomes and goals can be achieved, even though many of the interviewees did not feel this was currently the case.

Fourth, many of the interviewees were keen to advocate the need for a public health system to be based on good evidence or intelligence, rather than influenced by vested interests. For a public health system to be truly effective, several interviewees suggested that policies, targets and interventions ought to be more closely based on the available evidence and information at both local and national levels:

> PCT: One critical thing that underpins all of this, of course, is good, effective information systems and being able to analyse and understand the health needs of populations at a local level, because, without that, you can't create the arguments that will persuade people to change what they're doing.

The effective supply and use of information and evidence was seen by several interviewees to be particularly important in the light of recent moves to encourage joint commissioning for health and wellbeing. The interviewees' comments on the need for the use of evidence to be far better in public health planning and decision-making suggests that the post-1997 emphasis on evidence-based policy and practice (see Box 2.1) has not had as much impact as might have been hoped for.

Fifth, a number of the interviewees felt the system should reflect a public sector ethos, being publicly accountable and transparent and reflecting a number of other key values, including professionalism, value for money, respect for individual freedom, choice, having a long-term vision and an acceptance of the links between public health and some environmental values.

In addition to the significance of the above values to public health, interviewees placed considerable emphasis on leadership. The need for effective leadership within a public health system was articulated by a narrow majority of the interviewees and many of them expressed disappointment at the limited leadership within England's current public health system, at both national and local levels:

> SHA: I think we've lacked public health leadership. Public health got too focused on standards of practice and all sorts of inward-looking things ... Big changes to the health of the public and the determinants of the health of the public have been floating past its window, and all it's been really focused on are the standards of public health practice, and it's really missed the point.

The absence of leadership has become a familiar refrain within debates about public health, yet there appears to be a dearth of effective programmes aimed at remedying this deficit. The reasons for this ongoing disparity may lie in McAreavey et al's (2001: 460) assessment that: "further work is required to delineate what 'effective' public health leadership means both in relation to 'transformational' leadership characteristics ... and in relation to training and continuous professional development requirements". Yet, over time a clearer idea of what skills and attributes public health leaders require has emerged (Hunter, 2007b), suggesting there are now greater possibilities for addressing this issue than McAreavey and colleagues felt there were in 2001.

The final dimension of a desirable public health system reflected by our interviewees was the importance of enabling local flexibility in dealing with public health issues. Perhaps reinforced by multiple frustrations with central government's short-term outlook, but more overtly triggered by concerns with nationally enforced targets, several of the interviewees were keen to highlight the importance of having a public health system that could be adapted at a local level to meet the specific needs of different communities:

> NGO: Local freedom to do things is absolutely critical in public health because when I've seen good examples of how things work it's because they've emerged that way, not because somebody said, 'this is what you've got to do'.

These different strands are relevant for understanding how a public health system is constructed and understood by key stakeholders, and how different aspects of a public health system work together in practice.

Developing a public health system

As a specific example of support for the notion of a public health system in England, the North West Region has developed the concept following a workshop in which participants reflected on, and attempted to map, the public health system in order to explore its implications at a regional level (Ellis, 2005). The workshop report identified a number of issues that needed to be addressed to achieve a public health system that was 'fit for purpose' in this region:

- The overall public health system needs to be mapped and described: which organisations are part of it, and what each is required to contribute to improve and protect health.
- An organisation's contribution to public health should not be optional and it should be held accountable for its delivery.
- Organisational boundaries can be an obstacle to delivery – all relevant organisations should have a duty of partnership and should recognise the public health system will become network driven, with people contributing from all levels; the workforce must be liberated from its 'silos' to enable cross-skilling and provide public health input where the people who need it are located.
- To overcome the fragmentation in public health governance between district and regional levels and across different agencies, a more coherent and robust accountability structure is required.
- The subsidiarity principle should apply, namely, that the delivery of public health goals should be undertaken locally wherever possible, and be the responsibility of a jointly appointed DPH, accountable to the local authority and NHS; higher-tier (for example, regional) responsibility should be reserved for rare incidents and scarce expertise, and for developing strategic frameworks informed by those responsible for local delivery.
- The rate and number of innovative schemes is unsustainable, especially when they are subject to short-term funding and fail to get mainstreamed, even when demonstrably effective; more work needs to be put into (a) mainstreaming innovations that work by using real-time research and development that is both relevant and timely in meeting public health goals, and (b) acting on the evidence where appropriate.
- Greater health literacy is called for, as recommended, for example, by Wanless (2002); people need to be engaged in their health and understand what contributes to, and damages, it in order to help foster a form of advocacy and the creation of 'tipping points' whereby

pressure is put on government to act in the interests of the public good (Gladwell, 2001).

- Employers are a key platform for strengthening health literacy among the workforce and this is in keeping with the healthy settings approach advocated in the 1999 health strategy; as 49% of the North West GDP is spent in the public sector this should be an 'engine' for action on public health.
- Intelligence needs to be analysed at a higher level of aggregation and results should be locally accessible; all parts of a public health delivery system should be obliged to collect quality information so it can be analysed and acted on; vertical integration of the public health system is needed in respect of shared information systems, shared policy objectives at each level and high quality R&D.

Another attempt to embed a public health ethos across a wide range of sectors is evident in a study carried out in England for The King's Fund (Hunter and Marks, 2005). It promotes a notion of 'public health governance', placing significant emphasis on the 'stewardship' role of government and the development of 'proactive public health organisations'. Drawing parallels with corporate and clinical governance, Hunter and Marks suggest that 'public health governance' ought to embrace four dimensions: professional performance, resource use, risk management and public satisfaction with interventions/services. Furthermore, the authors argue: "public health governance must be rigorous in its application, organisation-wide in its emphasis, accountable in its delivery, developmental in its thrust, and positive in its impact" (Hunter and Marks, 2005: 43). In this conception, the development of public health governance is closely tied to the notion of 'proactive public health organisations'.

Such organisations:

- recognise that improving the public's health and reducing health inequalities is a proactive process – not a reactive one that deals with the consequences of ill health;
- recognise that this process goes beyond the NHS or any other, single actor;
- integrate policy streams and resource flows, so that suitable proactive public health policies can be crafted and implemented;
- make public health part of everybody's job description;
- 'complete the loop' by building public health needs into its monitoring and appraisal processes, so that successes and failures can be identified and adapted (Hunter and Marks, 2005: 44).

Rather than denoting the creation of a new organisation – and similar to the notions of creating a 'public health system' or focusing on 'capacity building' – the idea of proactive public health organisations involves embedding an ethos of public health into mainstream thinking so that all organisations of relevance to the public's health become 'proactive public health organisations'. Creating such organisations will require a commitment to change as well as the appropriate investment of resources.

Conclusion

While the above approaches each adopt a slightly different perspective on promoting public health, they share a commitment to developing a widespread culture of public health improvement across a range of sectors that regard themselves as part of a public health system and whose activities are aligned to achieve a common purpose. In our view, given the continuing problems over defining with any precision what public health is and who should do it, it would perhaps make more sense to have a clear understanding of the potential constituents of a public health system so that, when issues arise in public health, appropriate parts of that system can be mobilised. This might include policy advocacy as well as issues around governance and delivery. Such a pragmatic way forward might avoid the interminable and inconclusive debates over who practises public health and what specialist training they might need. Instead, it would not matter where practitioners and skill sets were located as long as there was an understanding that they formed part of a public health system and shared its underlying ethos and values.

THREE

The evolution of the public health function in England (1): 1974–97

Previous chapters have indicated the potential breadth of a public health system. Chapters Three and Four are devoted to providing a historical account of the public health function in England. This chapter takes 1974 as its starting point, which is when lead responsibility for public health was transferred from local government to the NHS, where it has remained ever since. It covers the period between this significant change and 1997, when there was a change of government, which had significant implications for public health policy. The next chapter picks up the story from 1997 to 2009.

The evolution of public health policy and practice in England since 1974 has been underpinned by a number of overlapping and recurring themes and schisms, several of which were described in the last chapter. Principal among these, and in no particular order, are the following:

- what constitutes public health policy and practice, and how the function (that is, the organisation with main responsibility) is defined;
- the optimal location of the public health function;
- the relationship between health improvement and inequalities in health;
- the population focus of public health vis-à-vis attempts to influence individual lifestyles;
- the nature and conceptualisation of the workforce, in terms of both capacity and capability;
- the nature and scope of the public health system;
- the balance between collective responsibility and individual choice;
- the balance between 'upstream' public health interventions and health care services;
- the extent to which primary care focuses on population health;
- public health's advocacy role in relation to its corporate identity (that is, activist versus 'technician-manager' roles) (Berridge, 2006: xxiii).

Debates about each of these issues have recurred in cyclical fashion during the evolution of the public health function since the 1970s and most remain contested and largely unresolved issues for current policy and practice. The first part of this chapter examines the rise of the new public health in the UK, which occurred in the late 1970s, and which encouraged practitioners and policy makers to focus on the wider health agenda and break free from a restrictive obsession with health care and ill health. The second part of the chapter provides a brief account of the main developments in the location and organisation of the public health function since 1974. There is an inevitable focus on the NHS and public health medicine because that is where, for better or worse, much of the attention and actions have centred in terms of policy and practice, and also where many of the power struggles around professional and practice issues have been played out. However, as is further discussed in Chapter Four, developments in local government, both through neighbourhood renewal and regeneration initiatives and through broad partnerships for health and wellbeing, have played an increasingly important role in framing a public health agenda (Stewart, 2007) and we have also sought to capture these developments. The final part of this chapter considers the extent to which 1974 marked a turning point in the fortunes of public health practitioners, setting the stage for a series of recurring debates.

Emergence of the new public health

From the late 1970s, tensions and reorganisations surrounding the public health function in England were concurrent with a broader, international movement that came to be known as the 'new public health'. This movement threw into relief the aridity and reductionist nature of narrow, professional debates. The period was also marked by a sense of growing exasperation among many involved in public health with the neglect of public health and preventive initiatives. These perceptions and developments were instrumental in fostering a broad, and some would say political, movement concerned to put in place what came to be known as 'the new public health'. This movement drew on the spirit of the early pioneers in public health but within the context of the new health challenges (Unit for the Study of Health Policy, 1979; Ashton and Seymour, 1988). Webster (1992: 10) argues that, "as in the 1930s, much of the impetus for the New Public Health has emerged from outside the ranks of public health organisations, initiatives in other western nations, or lay and scientific pressure groups". The movement also reflected critiques of the scope of clinical medicine in improving population health when compared with the impact of better nutrition and healthier environments (McKeown, 1976) and an emerging body of literature that underlined the interplay between health and social and environmental factors, and emphasised the role of public policy, intersectoral collaboration and community action. As such, it prefigures later attempts to interpret and define a broad public health system. A key influence was the publication of a Canadian policy document called *A new perspective on the health of Canadians* (Lalonde, 1974), which became known as 'the Lalonde report', after the Minister of Health and Welfare at the time, Marc Lalonde. This report with its concept of four health fields (environment, human biology, lifestyle and health care organisation) quickly received international attention and acclaim for its persuasive arguments concerning the need to shift the focus of health policy from health care to the prevention of ill health.

Despite the difficulties arising for public health from the national political context in England during the 1980s – a period marked by a retrenchment in public spending and an ethos that resisted spending on ambitious public programmes to tackle social and health issues – it was a fertile period of progressive advances for public health at regional and international levels, supported by links between the two, as a witness seminar on public health in England recounts (Evans and Knight, 2006). The WHO conference at Alma Ata in 1978 (WHO, 1978) was followed by the WHO's *Health for All by the Year 2000* policy (WHO, 1981) and the Ottawa Charter for Health Promotion in 1986 (WHO, 1986). The Ottawa Charter is often considered to have been ahead of its time and its full importance and potential have yet to be fully realised (Hills and McQueen, 2007). These seminal reports emphasised the importance of healthy public policy, community action and supportive environments as well as the personal skills involved in making healthy choices. Such approaches were increasingly adopted by health promotion officers and others who, at that time, presented a radical and alternative approach to the public health establishment (Berridge et al, 2006). There was a link between the emerging 'new public health', with its interest in participation, and the community health movement, which was promoting a commitment to empowerment, informed action and capacity building. Community health needs assessment began to incorporate equity and socio-environmental issues, and moved towards a more participatory approach, attempting to understand, rather than merely describe, health needs. Despite the Thatcher government's uncomfortable stance towards health promotion, particular English regions were highly focused on developing public health during the 1980s. Liverpool, which produced one of England's first regional reports on public health (Ashton, 1984), was a notable example. In this context, international links between various regional public health projects developed, such as those between Liverpool and North Karelia in Finland (Berridge et al, 2006).

The 'Healthy Cities' project, first established by WHO in 1985, was viewed as a test bed for *Health for All*. It was thought that strategies for building supportive environments, combating health inequalities and developing healthy public policies could be created and evaluated at city level so that real change could take place. The 'Healthy Cities' initiative was probably more successful as a concept than as practical reality, especially since the freedoms enjoyed by local authorities in the UK were limited. Nevertheless, 'Healthy Cities' projects endeavoured to develop intersectoral collaboration between local authorities, health services, voluntary agencies and the private sector.

The new public health movement in the UK in the mid-1980s was partly aimed at recreating the link between environmental health and public health medicine, which had been severed by the 1974 NHS reorganisation and the transfer of public health medicine (see section below). Ashton and Seymour's (1988) book, with its title *The new public health*, quickly became a landmark publication. The authors saw "health promotion as the means to health for all", by which they meant "a process of enabling people to increase control over and improve their health" (Ashton and Seymour, 1988: 25). The impact of the environment and a wide range of social factors on health was regarded as supremely important by public health organisations such as the Public Health Alliance, whose Charter for Public Health published in 1987 (Upward, 1998) included environmental change in respect of housing, food and work – commitments now reflected in the work of the UKPHA (2007) with its pledge to promote sustainable development and challenge a wide range of anti-health forces. Environmental protection was also perceived to be critical to public health and concern was expressed that, with the loss of local medical officers of health, environmental protection measures had been downgraded in importance.

As has been well documented, concerns about growing inequalities in health and the role played by poverty and social conditions in determining health were largely ignored by the Thatcher administration (Berridge and Blume, 2003). The Black Report (Department of Health and Social Security, 1980), which had been established by a Labour government but reported to a Conservative one, argued that social inequalities in health were largely the result of material-structuralist factors. However, its findings had little impact on policy and the report was effectively shelved (although it did have a big impact on the public health community and the international and regional developments described above). Although arguments were put forward in this era for a multidisciplinary approach to public health and health promotion (for example, Unit for the Study of Health Policy, 1979) and for the establishment of consultant-level posts from backgrounds other than medicine, these developments did not become reality until many years later.

It is in this context that, in 1987, after it had produced a series of rather critical reports, the semi-independent Health Education Council (which had replaced the Central Council for Health Education in 1967) was supplanted by the markedly less independent special health authority, the Health Education Authority (for the background to this change, see Sutherland, 1987). In time, health promotion became less concerned with a social ecological approach to public health and retreated back to a focus on individual lifestyles and behaviour change.

At the same time as these national and international developments for a new public health were gathering momentum, tensions persisted over the nature, organisation and location of the public health workforce in England.

The organisation of the public health function in England post-1974

In this section, we reflect on the recurring tensions that have characterised the development of public health since the mid-1970s: first, in relation to the organisation of public health and the pressures on it; second, in terms of the divide between primary care and public health; and, finally, in the development of a multidisciplinary workforce. This account demonstrates how the public health system in England has been incrementally pieced together, almost by default.

Public health under pressure

In the period between 1974 and 1997, most major public health responsibilities were transferred from local government to the NHS (although this did not affect all services of importance to health and, notably, responsibility for environmental health remained with local government). This was followed by a long and chequered process of attempting to ensure that responsibility for public health was shared between agencies and across locations, with a truly multidisciplinary workforce being the aim.

Our story begins with the demise of the medical officers of health (MOsH) and the shift of much of their work from the local authority to the NHS. Support for change grew in 1970 and 1972 when social work and environmental health were respectively each separated from the MOsH's responsibilities, thereby weakening their influence. Also in 1972, following a recommendation of the Todd Commission on Medical Education which reported in 1968 (Todd Commission, 1968), the Faculty for Community Medicine was established, with membership restricted to registered medical practitioners. It is in this context that, at the time of the 1974 NHS reorganisation, public health changed its name to 'community medicine' and was integrated into the NHS. This transition meant that the MOsH and the public health department disappeared, with the majority of MOsH becoming 'community physicians' appointed by the NHS. As noted above, responsibility for environmental health remained with local government under directors of environmental health.

The role of 'community physicians', as originally conceived by Morris (1969), revolved around a concern with epidemiology and population health. However, as a witness seminar in London testified (Berridge et al, 2006), there was a great deal of confusion as to what the role of community physicians involved. A survey of community physicians (with service roles) in English health authorities undertaken by the King's Fund Institute demonstrated that there was considerable uncertainty about lines of accountability and, furthermore, that there was evidence of gaps in training and skills, especially around environmental health and communicable disease control, as well as potential tensions around the advisory role of community physicians to local authorities (Harvey and Judge, 1988). Another survey of community physicians in England showed that 60% of their time was taken up with administration and only 9% with preventive medicine (Donaldson and Hall, 1979). Stewart (1987: 734) sums up some of the frustrations of this period:

> [The role of specialists in community medicine was] never clearly defined or understood even within the specialty and, lacking in executive and infrastructural clout, was further eroded by subsequent reorganisations. In many health authorities, the specialist in community medicine now operates alone, without a department, with equivocal status, and a self-made or uncertain range of duties which are often seen to be marginal or trivial even when there is room for individual initiative.

Stewart (1987: 736) goes on to claim that the range of job titles and responsibilities within the field of 'community medicine' was unclear, arguing: "Designations are useless unless they describe the job in a manner understandable to medical and non-medical colleagues and to the public". It is a view that remains alive in more recent discussions about public health. For example, McPherson et al (1999: 4) claim that public health has long suffered from being "too close to health care and too far from health", by which they mean that public health has been "largely administered from within the NHS and the focus of resources has tended to be on individual patient care at the expense of public health activities targeted at the wider population"(McPherson et al, 1999: 4). Given that health services are demand led and public health policy led, they conclude that the former will continue to attract the lion's share of resources, "whatever the rational merits of the situation" (McPherson et al, 1999: 26). This view is echoed by many of those who gave evidence to the Health Committee's public health inquiry in 2001 (House of Commons Health Committee, 2001a, 2001b).

As Hunter (2003) notes, community medicine appears to have encountered two major problems in trying to fulfil Morris's original vision: first, their location within the health service separated community physicians from many of the relevant factors and agencies that they were trying to work with (for example, housing, employment and environment); second, community physicians' concern with collective population health often brought them into conflict with the individualised focus of other medical practitioners. Indeed, as the discussions at two witness seminars both indicated (Berridge et al, 2006; Evans and Knight, 2006), the community physicians of the 1980s were not accorded the same respect as consultants in other medical specialities, leading to tensions between the Faculty for Public Health and the British Medical Association. The fact that there was (and remains) no trade union specifically for public health workers in England may have further hindered progress towards a multidisciplinary workforce.

Since 1974, when local government was stripped of many of its public health responsibilities, many believe that the public health profession was hijacked by a managerialist agenda focused on health care services and that it became part of an essentially NHS agenda, which was more concerned with downstream, secondary and largely hospital-based care than upstream measures of primary prevention. It has been argued that, post-1974, insufficient attention was given to local social and environmental determinants of health by specialists in community medicine. Webster (2002) claims that community medicine's limited success was reflected in its failure to reshape the health service in favour of health prevention and promotion. Instead, it presided over the increasing fragmentation of public health responsibilities and activities. Berridge (1999) notes the unease among community physicians about their loss of contact with the local community and their increasing role in managing health services, rather than analysing broader health problems. Lewis (1986) goes further and suggests:

> The position of community physicians was subject to serious conflicts in terms both of their relationship with other members of the medical profession, and the nature of their primary responsibility, whether for the management of health services or for the analysis of health problems and health needs. (Lewis, 1986: 135)

She concludes that the role of community physicians was very much determined by their place in the new NHS.

While many in public health were concerned about the downstream focus of much of their work within the NHS, others accepted it as the price to be paid for securing a seat at the top table when it came to deciding how resources should be allocated and priorities agreed. Nevertheless, as Webster (2002) points out, community medicine failed to achieve the status intended by its architects and recruitment declined.

Yet, despite some claims to the contrary, it is important to acknowledge that there has never been a 'golden age' in public health, even though there is a widespread perception that things were somehow better pre-1974, when public health was a local government responsibility led by the MOsH, who were often key figures in their communities. As Lewis (1986) notes, while MOsH, being separate from the NHS, could in theory consider the health of the entire community rather than simply concern themselves with health service considerations, they rarely did so in practice. As she goes on to say: "it cannot be argued that the transition to community medicine was achieved at the expense of an enormously vigorous public health system" (Lewis, 1986: 163). However, MOsH did have formal authority to investigate any factor with a bearing on health and had security of tenure, which meant that they could criticise employing authorities with impunity (Editorial, 1981). There were examples of inspired leadership where effective MOsH displayed networking skills and personal diplomacy of relevance to contemporary public health, especially in the context of partnership working (Gorsky, 2007). Such leadership also involved facing down vested interests, thereby combining social conscience with scientific intent. In the end, the failure of MOsH had much to do with the orientation of the NHS towards the hospital service and the attenuation of local authority powers, which served to marginalise public health, demoralise the profession and deprive it of resources. As Gorsky points out: "soon after 1974, fears that something had been lost with the MOH began to be articulated" (Gorsky, 2007: 471).

Concerns about the public health profession and practice go far beyond its optimal location and certainly predate 1974, although they have come to a head since then. In her account of public health since 1919, Lewis (1986: 3) claims that the most important failure of public health "was its lack of a firm philosophy to guide it in approaching health problems". Such a state of affairs has continued to the present day with fluid notions of public health alternating between a focus on personal prevention and a focus on structural determinants, enshrined in the notion of healthy public policy. Moreover, public health professionals throughout this period have continued to occupy a subservient position within the medical profession. Moves in recent years to open up public health to those who are not clinically qualified have done little to dent this deep-seated power imbalance. Lewis argues that the vacuum created by the lack of a coherent philosophy was the principal reason for some observers suggesting that public health resembled a 'ragbag of activities', unconnected by any guiding principles. It could be argued that it was not so much the absence of a unifying theory that was the problem as the existence of several competing theories, each with its respective advocates and lobbyists, both inside and outside the public health system. Which is ascendant depends on the prevailing political and ideological context.

For whatever reason, the absence of a clearly articulated and widely accepted philosophy and set of values underpinning the public health function remains a concern in establishing and sustaining a vigorous public health system, as described in the previous chapter. It may also account for the continuing fragility and vulnerability of the public health profession, which has been a consistent feature throughout its development but especially so since 1974, from which point onwards the focus and direction of public health has been inextricably tied to the NHS. Some of the above observations concerning the state of public health during the 20th century in England are echoed in Julio Frenk's important essay on the international crisis in public health, published some years later in 1992, in which he wrote:

> ... public health has historically been one of the vital forces leading to reflection on, and collective action for, health and well-being. The widespread impression exists today, however, that this leading role has been weakening and that public health is experiencing a severe identity crisis, as well as a crisis of organisation and accomplishment. (Frenk, 1992: 68)

In the UK, under the post-1979 Thatcher government, a series of organisational reforms in the NHS further affected those involved in public health (see Appendix for details of the changing structures). First, in 1980–82, there was a reorganisation from area health authorities to district health authorities (DHAs), which was followed by the gradual introduction of the internal market to the NHS, between 1989 and 1991. For the public health workforce, the introduction of the internal market meant new opportunities for some people (associated with a renewed interest in population health resulting from the commissioning role of some parts of the NHS) but severe marginalisation for others, especially those working in health promotion (Evans and Knight, 2006). Organisations such as the Public Health Alliance (established in 1987) emerged as various individuals and networks attempted to keep the community development and health promotion aspects of public health alive. While they did important work, these efforts remained overshadowed by the continuing pull of the NHS and acute care sector, neither of which was primarily concerned with prevention.

During this period, various outbreaks of diseases called attention to the necessity of a public health strategy in England. As well as the emergence of new communicable diseases, such as HIV/AIDS, there was a series of high-profile food health scares, including outbreaks of salmonella poisoning and the emergence of BSE/CJD. The lack of clarity of workforce responsibilities following the reforms in the early 1980s, along with a shift towards a focus on chronic disease, were seen as contributory factors in several major communicable disease outbreaks later that decade, including the Stanley Royd Hospital outbreak of salmonellosis (Department of Health and Social Security, 1986). Eventually, the various crises in 'community medicine' and 'public health' led to an official inquiry into the public health function in England, led by the Chief Medical Officer of the time, Donald Acheson. The critical nature of much of the evidence presented to this inquiry underlines the extent to which dissatisfaction had grown. For example, the Department of Community Health at the London School of Hygiene and Tropical Medicine stated:

> Achievement of the fundamental tasks of community medicine is often frustrated. This is for a number of reasons including the short-term perspective of management in the NHS; the lack of non-medical members in community medicine teams; a shortage of support staff and facilities; the underdevelopment of the necessary tools for evaluating interventions; and inadequate continuing education facilities. (Department of Community Health [unpublished], 1986: 1)

The Department of Community Health's evidence also contends that community medicine suffered from a lack of sufficient knowledge and skills to carry out fundamental tasks, and experienced some antagonism from medically qualified staff towards the advent of multidisciplinary teams. It further notes concern with the recruitment of doctors to community medicine: "It is our contention that a major factor that has deterred potential recruits has been the lack of a clear image of the role and tasks involved" (Department of Community Health [unpublished], 1986: 11). Other evidence submitted to the inquiry included a report from the Institution of Environmental Health Officers (also unpublished), which claimed that local authorities might be a more appropriate location for the public health function than health authorities. A common thread throughout the various submissions was the confusion surrounding the role and function of community physicians.

The resulting publication of Acheson's (1988) inquiry outlined the need for a multidisciplinary approach to public health, while simultaneously reinforcing the assumption that the discipline should be led by medical professionals (with other professions playing no more than a supportive role). It was on the recommendation of this report that community medicine was renamed public health medicine. The report also highlighted a shortage in consultants in health protection and recommended an initial workforce target of 15.8 specialists per million of the population. While the report endorsed the WHO's *Health for All* strategy, its recommendations were criticised as "over-influenced by the self interests of community physicians and environmental health officers", ignoring the role of the public and of the voluntary sector (Ashton, 1988: 232).

In the structure that emerged, although directors of public health were supported by multidisciplinary teams, there were significant tensions in terms of the inequalities of opportunities for non-medical staff working within this system, which led some of those involved to set up their own *ad hoc* networks (Evans and Knight, 2006). However, these networks did not have professional status and, furthermore, the career structures for non-medical public health staff were extremely limited, with existing training and career development pathways focusing exclusively on those who were medically qualified. The extent of the increasing frustration among non-medically qualified staff at the lack of career prospects open to them is vividly apparent in the discussions at a 2006 witness seminar on the origins and development of multidisciplinary public health in the UK (Evans and Knight, 2006).

Across the great divide: public health and primary care

A further long-standing problem, noted in Chapter One, has been the organisational divide between public health and primary care, the latter typically identified with GP practice, notwithstanding the breadth of the Declaration of Alma Ata. This has given rise to problems between many GPs and public health practitioners over the years. The medical model underpinning many definitions of primary care (and public health for that matter) has inhibited the development of community perspectives on health (Taylor et al, 1998). The 1946 NHS Act did not include prevention in the contract for GPs, a situation that continued until the late 1970s when the Royal College of GPs took up the cause of prevention and 'anticipatory care'. Lewis (1987) points out, for example, that GPs were suspicious of the aims of MOsH in the 1960s to build health centres, which would allow them to coordinate community-based health services. She quotes Titmuss (1965), who asked whether there would be a place for the MOH and the public health department if GPs were to become community doctors. Despite interest in anticipatory care, this largely meant individually oriented, *clinical* anticipatory care. There has been a steady stream of influential GPs who have argued for primary care to exploit its public health potential (Pickles, 1929; Fry, 1968; Tudor Hart, 1988) and to demonstrate a greater commitment to promoting the health of the local population. Many argued the public health content of primary care needed to be recognised and made explicit and Mant and Anderson (1985) claimed, for example, that it made sense for community medicine and general practice to move towards integration. They pointed out the ironies of "the divisions in the structure of the health service which have led to a community-medicine specialty without access to the community and a primary-health-care system without responsibility for the community's health" (Mant and Anderson, 1985: 1114). Others also argued that public health had to recognise both approaches, even though they were organised and funded in different ways (Stone, 1987).

Towards a multidisciplinary workforce

Throughout the period under review, the public health profession remained equated with public health medicine, with other relevant groups often being defined by the description 'non-medical' (Evans, 2003). However, in 1991, the publication of *The nation's health* underlined a growing acceptance in policy terms that the public health function should not be defined by, or restricted to, a medical specialty (Jacobson et al, 1991). With increasing calls to develop a multidisciplinary public health workforce, resulting from a combination of 'top down' and 'bottom up' pressures (Evans and Knight, 2006), some university public health postgraduate courses began to attract non-medically qualified students. Following the establishment of the first multidisciplinary Master of Public Health (MPH) degrees at Cardiff University in 1990, the Master of Public Health at the London School of Hygiene and Tropical Medicine became the first equivalent course in England to allow students from disciplines other than medicine to enrol in 1992. However, what the career opportunities for the newly qualified non-medical MPH graduates would be remained rather unclear. Although the Conservative government's *The Health of the Nation* strategy (Secretary of State for Health, 1992), the first of its kind in England, signalled a shift towards a public health focus, it was almost solely concerned with health promotion, failing to acknowledge a need to tackle wider socio-economic and environmental determinants of health or to deal seriously with the dominance of health care services within the NHS (Department of Health, 1998a; Hunter, 2003).

As concern to highlight the multidisciplinary nature of public health grew, a postal survey of public health professionals in 1994 identified over 1,000 people from non-medical backgrounds working in public health in the UK (Somervaille and Griffiths, 1995). This information fed into the establishment of a working group to explore this issue, which was followed by a series of annual national seminars in Birmingham to explore career structures and training and accreditation requirements for multidisciplinary roles in public health. In 1996, following one of these national conferences, concerned individuals established the Multi-disciplinary Public Health Forum (MDPHF), which aimed to promote the multidisciplinary nature of public health and the associated training needs. In 1997, a joint statement of intent was issued by the MDPHF and the Royal Institute of Public Health that they would work together on the development of a framework for education, development and accreditation of multidisciplinary public health professionals.

Conclusion

As this chapter has endeavoured to show, the developments evident in the new public health in the mid-1980s, both in the UK and internationally, have had limited impact on the public health function, thereby testifying to its limitations and narrow outlook. Instead of seizing the opportunities offered by the new public health to raise the importance of public health on the policy agenda, the function was largely preoccupied by its own position and status, particularly in regard to what might be termed its special relationship with the NHS. Although this relationship was regarded as essential to maintaining the credibility of the function in the eyes of the medical profession, it prevented those working within it from being liberated enough to think actively about public health in broader, non-medical ways. This cleavage remains a live issue today, as the next chapter shows.

FOUR

The evolution of the public health function in England (2): 1997–2009

The election of the New Labour government in 1997 represented an important shift for public health, or so it seemed, as the party had made bold and ambitious commitments to tackling health inequalities and addressing the wider determinants of health in its election manifesto. A series of documents and debates stressing the need to give higher priority to the health of the public, to end the fragmentation of the public health function and to start seriously developing and strengthening its multidisciplinary nature subsequently emerged (Department of Health, 1998a, 1998b; Secretary of State for Health, 1999). The decade or so since 1997 has been a particularly active and fertile period for public health, although many of the issues at stake are familiar and have their antecedents in the period reviewed in Chapter Three. It has also been a somewhat chaotic and turbulent period, marked by numerous policy initiatives and structural changes, many of which appear to lack coherence. A number of these changes were not directed primarily at the public health function but their impacts have nevertheless been profound and are still being worked through. Some public health functions were relocated to arm's length bodies, a network of stand-alone organisations that include the National Institute for Health and Clinical Excellence (NICE) and the Health Protection Agency (HPA). Box 4.1 charts the changing organisational context for health protection.

Box 4.1: Health protection on the move

Health protection is largely concerned with infectious disease control, chemical and radiological hazards, emergency planning and the health care response to emergencies, including bioterrorism. In recent years, health protection has undergone significant change in respect of its organisation and location. The division of responsibilities for key public health functions was altered with the publication of *Getting ahead of the curve* (Department of Health, 2002), which created the HPA. This new agency, which was established to provide expertise on potential health threats such as infections and toxic hazards, took over much of the responsibility for public health protection. The creation of the HPA was the culmination of a number of changes in the nature and location of the health protection workforce starting in the mid-1970s.

Following recommendations made by the Inquiry into the Future of the Public Health Function (Acheson Report) in 1988, responsibility for public health and health protection passed to directors of public health (DsPH) in district health authorities (DHAs), supported by specialists in communicable disease and their teams. With the 2002 NHS reorganisation, these responsibilities passed to DsPH in primary care trusts (PCTs), supported by consultants in communicable disease control and performance managed by DsPH in strategic health authorities. Problems of the dispersal of responsibilities (as a result of the transfer from about 100 DHAs to over 300 PCTs) were addressed a year later by bringing together national expertise (for England and Wales) in the new HPA in 2003. The HPA provides advice and support to the NHS, local authorities, the Department of Health and others. It operates at national, regional and local levels and has absorbed the Public Health Laboratory Service, the National Poisons Information Service, the Centre for Applied Microbiology and Research, the National Focus for Chemical Incidents, the National Radiological Protection Board and all NHS public health staff responsible for health protection. It also became the location for consultants in disease control, with the exception of some of the community infection control staff who are based in PCTs.

The creation of the HPA has not overcome all of the perceived difficulties relating to health protection. In particular, disputes remain about the demarcation of the boundaries of health protection and the resulting accountability structures (Pickles, 2004). In a study of variation in the interpretation of health protection arrangements between PCTs and local health protection teams, Cosford et al (2006) point to problems arising from the shift from the provision of health protection through a single organisation, the DHAs (which was the case until 2002), to the new dual statutory responsibilities for PCTs and the HPA. As they highlight, this shift has resulted in some confusion; while PCTs are still responsible for community control of communicable disease and non-infectious environmental hazards, local arrangements for holding the HPA to account are based on a Memorandum of Understanding, which has no legal or statutory basis. Furthermore, the ways in which it is implemented vary across England, partly as a result of the skills gap in health protection. The researchers demonstrated a number of health protection functions (five out of 18) where there was a lack of consistency and concordance between participants and between organisations. These were:

- delivery of MMR vaccination following a student outbreak;
- infection control in private sector nursing homes;
- monitoring rates of sexually transmitted infections;
- immunisation training programmes for primary care staff;
- investigation of an apparent cluster of congenital abnormalities.

It has also been claimed that, while PCT public health teams are increasingly deskilled in health protection, formal accountability remains with the PCT and not with the HPA (personal communication). Perhaps not surprisingly, Pat Troop, the first chief executive officer (CEO) of the HPA, while acknowledging the "tensions and setbacks" surrounding the setting up of the Agency, defended its overall record, claiming that it "enabled us to identify the gaps in evidence, move to more consistent delivery, and create teams with greater critical mass for more effective responses and proactive programmes beyond managing outbreaks of infectious diseases" (Troop, 2007: 9). She also claimed that bringing together Agency staff with front-line practitioners was "beginning to demonstrate new ways of tackling old problems" and is, consequently, facilitating "a co-ordinated national response to major emergencies" (Troop, 2007: 9).

Strong views on the best location for health protection were expressed by a number of our interviewees, even though we did not ask specifically about this issue. One considered that the setting up of the HPA had been a "mistake", particularly in terms of what this meant for local services, as s/he felt that service delivery had been adversely affected as a result of the growing distance between the local level and the HPA.

This respondent favoured bringing the health protection domain back, not just into the NHS but to where it was pre-1974, which was "jointly with local authorities". Another interviewee commented that the HPA boundaries were often different from other boundaries, which caused problems with the moves towards greater coterminosity between NHS-based and other services.

Looking to the future of health protection, the same CEO claimed that health protection was much more in the public's eye and had a much higher media profile than previously (Troop, 2007). Troop believed this had implications for the continuing relevance of the Faculty's three public health domains. In particular, she argued that few public health problems did not require an element of all three domains and, moreover, that none "really encapsulates the structural, societal or international responses that are needed if we are to make progress. Nor do they capture the multi-agency nature of the work" (Troop, 2007: 9). Like others, her view is that a better way of conceptualising public health, and, indeed, the public

> health system, may be "to consider the range of knowledge, skills and techniques that are needed – in terms of tools that apply to all aspects of public health albeit with a different emphasis in different situations" (Troop, 2007: 9).
>
> Despite difficulties over the HPA's relationships with others charged with health protection responsibilities, a situation exacerbated by constant churn and organisational change within the NHS, there is probably general agreement that tackling the big issues around health protection demands a multi-levelled response, including national and international levels, and that a body like the HPA is therefore essential, even though it cannot deliver health protection alone but must work in partnership with other relevant bodies (Nicoll, 2007).

In what follows, we provide a brief overview in chronological order of the major policy and organisational changes that have occurred since 1997, which gives an indication of the changing topography of the policy and organisational landscape. We then describe their implications for the public health workforce and the objective of strengthening its multidisciplinary nature. As we concluded in Chapter Three, little progress had been achieved on this front prior to 1997. Since then, however, there have been a number of important developments, although how far these will truly succeed in gaining recognition for, and acceptance of, a multidisciplinary public health workforce remains to be seen. There has been greater emphasis on these issues over the past decade or so in response to perceived weaknesses in the evidence concerning particular interventions and in their effective implementation. A final section brings together some concluding observations from both this and the last chapter. It sets the scene for a discussion of the key issues that have come to the fore in recent debates about public health policy and practice, which forms the subject of Chapter Five.

The changing policy and organisational landscape in England

The period since 1997 has witnessed many important policy developments and changes in the management of public services, including an emphasis on joined-up working (that is, partnerships), which have contributed to local government being seen to have an increasingly significant public health role. There have also been developments around the organisation and delivery of health protection, a growing emphasis on the importance of the evidence base underpinning health interventions and increasingly extensive commitments to the use of targets in the performance management of policies and services. The period is also notable for a series of other major policy developments, including the impact of political devolution in the UK, with all that this implies for increasing divergence in health policies and structures (Greer and Rowland (eds), 2007; Greer, 2008). At the same time, and contributing to the growing policy divergence evident across the UK, within England there has been a strong push towards developing a market-style ethos in the NHS, with a focus on competition and choice. This has been accompanied by a renewed emphasis on commissioning for health and an expressed desire for more active public involvement. While these developments are not all aimed principally at public health, they have important implications for the function.

Major initiatives following the arrival of the New Labour government in May 1997 included the appointment of the first ever Minister for Public Health in 1997, the production of a new health strategy to replace *The Health of the Nation*, an independent assessment of the impact of *The Health of the Nation* (Department of Health, 1998a) and the establishment of an 'independent' inquiry into inequalities in health (chaired by Donald Acheson, a former Chief Medical Officer (CMO) for England) who had led the inquiry into the public health function in 1988. The Acheson Report (Acheson, 1998) made 39 recommendations for tackling health inequalities, the vast majority of which stretched far beyond the remit of the NHS. In the same year, an interim report of the *Chief Medical Officer's Project to Strengthen the Public Health Function*, mentioned in previous chapters, expressed a commitment to multidisciplinary working (Department of Health, 1998b).

In 1999, a new health strategy to replace *The Health of the Nation* was published, *Saving Lives: Our Healthier Nation* (Secretary of State for Health, 1999). It had been preceded a year earlier by a consultative document, which many working in public health considered to be a better document from a broader public health perspective (for example, Fulop and Hunter, 1999). In particular, the insertion of the first two words, 'saving lives', into the title seemed to signal that the strategy would remain firmly located within a health care model, with less emphasis on supporting communities to remain healthy and more on keeping individuals alive (Fulop and Hunter, 1999). Moreover, the strategy focused mainly on disease-based themes, despite criticisms that this represented an overly narrow, reductionist view of public health. As we outlined in Chapter One, this approach was predicated on a deficit model of health rather than an assets-oriented one, despite the fact that two independent assessments of the impact of *The Health of the Nation*, combined in a single published report, had demonstrated that the strategy's domination "by a disease-based approach" that was 'heavily 'medically led'…was a cause for concern among those local authorities which believed that they contributed more to a health agenda in its broadest sense than health authorities" (Department of Health, 1998a: 14). It was suggested that, in the case of the new health strategy, a sound and logical argument could be made for local government rather than the NHS taking the lead role in local implementation. Indeed, such a view was advanced in the Local Government Association (LGA) and UK Public Health Association's (UKPHA's) joint response to *Saving Lives: Our Healthier Nation* (LGA and UKPHA, 2000). These organisations concluded that the government's actual strategy amounted to little more than "the traditional concerns of public health medicine" and gave too little attention to the need to integrate local planning mechanisms in order to achieve truly joint strategies for health improvement. Indeed, very little progress was made on this front until the *Tackling health inequalities: A programme for action* initiative in 2003 (Department of Health, 2003a) (see later in this chapter).

In many respects, the more radical aspects of the government's early strategic thinking around public health, which gave it a significant leadership role, were subsequently overshadowed by the *NHS Plan*, published in 2000 (Department of Health, 2000). By this point, the NHS had risen back up the policy agenda and concern over waiting lists and times, the quality of care and a perception that NHS management was weak began to dominate the discussions about health policy, both inside government and in the media. The laudable intention to put health before health care began to fade and traditional health care delivery issues came to dominate ministerial attention once again. Indeed, the *NHS Plan* proved to be the first of an outpouring of policy redirection, advice and guidance, which appears to have continued, largely unabated, ever since.

The *NHS Plan*'s aim was to modernise the NHS and it outlined an ambitious ten-year strategy for doing so. With its principal focus on health care, public health did not figure prominently. Indeed, the issue was confined to a slim chapter, buried deep inside the Plan. There was, however, an emphasis on improved partnership working and cross-government action, and new local strategic partnerships were announced. The other important development was the announcement of national targets for reducing health inequalities in 2001, which were subsequently revised into a single target on health inequalities in 2002, namely, by 2010 to reduce inequalities in health outcomes by 10% as measured by infant mortality and life expectancy at birth (HM Treasury, 2002). Previously, the government had resisted setting such targets, leaving the matter to local discretion. The *NHS Plan* also announced the introduction of new single, integrated public health groups across NHS regional offices and government offices of the regions. These forums were intended to encourage an approach to neighbourhood renewal and regeneration that combined social and economic development with health concerns.

The *NHS Plan* was regarded as the apotheosis of a command and control style of policy making and, as such, was heavily criticised. The government was accused of 'control freakery' and of adopting a highly centralised style of management, which was deemed wholly inappropriate. In response, the government did an unexpected volte-face, announcing a major shift in the balance of power from centre to periphery in 2001 (Department of Health, 2001d). These changes plunged the NHS into yet another extensive upheaval and ushered in a period of instability and uncertainty, which ended only with the next major restructuring commencing in 2005. The *Shifting the Balance of Power* (STBOP) (Department of Health, 2001d) changes served to distract attention from implementing the *NHS Plan* as employees worried about their future jobs. The centrepiece of the STBOP changes introduced in 2003 was the primary care trusts (PCTs), which were to assume control over 75% of the NHS budget as well as responsibility for commissioning care for their local populations. Each PCT board had to appoint a director of public health. The location of directorates of public health in PCTs and the formation of public health networks to cross organisational boundaries could be seen as encouraging the long-standing division between primary health care and public health that is described in Chapter Three.

The other key development as far as public health was concerned was its strengthening at regional level. This entailed replacing the existing eight NHS regional offices with four new health and social care regions. In fact the four regions were soon disbanded and their functions absorbed by the strategic health authorities (SHAs), but the regional directors of public health (RDsPH) largely remained located within the regional government offices (although at least one RDPH has relocated himself to the SHA). Although the move of regional public health into the government offices was widely welcomed on the basis that it was hoped a strong health component could be built into regional programmes in areas such as transport, environment and urban regeneration, there remained doubts over whether the public health function, as currently configured, would be able to meet the challenge.

Moreover, there was no option but to fill RDPH posts with medically qualified personnel, since the role combined local government office duties with those of medical director.

Reflecting a more widespread concern that public health was failing to receive the attention it both deserved and had been promised by the incoming Labour government, the House of Commons Health Committee launched an inquiry into public health in 2000. Its terms of reference were "to examine the co-ordination between central government, local government, health authorities and PCGs [primary care groups]/PCTs in promoting and delivering public health" (House of Commons Health Committee, 2001a: xii). In the course of its inquiry, the Committee examined a number of initiatives, including health action zones (for a discussion of these see Box 4.2), healthy living centres and health improvement programmes, the role and status of the Minister of Public Health (which was allegedly downgraded following the departure of the first post-holder) and the role of the Director of Public Health (DPH). With such wide-ranging terms of reference and only limited time (under a year) to produce its report, the Committee could not do justice to the full complexities of the subject but nevertheless made a brave attempt. In addition to the main report, the inquiry resulted in a considerable amount of evidence, which was published in a second, accompanying, volume to the main report (House of Commons Health Committee, 2001b). The Health Committee was critical of government health policy and its focus on health care, concluding that policy approaches were out of kilter with much expert opinion and with the government's own early commitment to shifting the policy agenda from a preoccupation with health care to one more committed to health improvement and wellbeing. In its view, 'fix and mend' medical services continued to receive the major share of attention and resources, and there remained profound systemic and structural problems with joined-up working, which went beyond the mere absence of incentives to collaborate. The Committee also expressed concern that the *NHS Plan* represented a lost opportunity to give a real boost to public health and that the health strategy, *Saving Lives*, had been somewhat marginalised by it.

Box 4.2: Health action zones

Introduced in 1997, health action zones (HAZs) were one of New Labour's 'flagship' area-based policies, which were intended to address some of the new government's public health commitments, particularly reducing health inequalities. The initiative was independently evaluated and has therefore been well documented (Bauld et al, 2001, 2005; Burton and Diaz de Leon, 2002; Kane, 2002; Sullivan et al, 2002, 2004; Benzeval, 2003; Bonner, 2003; Halliday and Asthana, 2005). The areas that were designated HAZ status varied significantly in terms of both geographical and population size and the number of organisational boundaries that they encompassed. It is therefore extremely difficult to define HAZs in any detail, but one of the main mechanisms that HAZs were expected to employ to achieve the public health goals set for them was to encourage effective partnership working, both between different organisations and sectors and between HAZ organisations and the local population. Nevertheless, HAZs often took very different approaches to achieving these goals, with some focusing on specific projects and others emphasising strategic changes in the way organisations within the HAZ worked, particularly in relation to their partnership with other actors. In total, 29 local areas were successful in their bid to be designated an HAZ (11 HAZs commenced in April 1998 and a further 15 in April 1999) but, in some cases, HAZs shared no more than the ability to access the extra resources set aside for them and an expectation that these resources would be employed to develop new and innovative ways of improving local population health outcomes and reducing health inequalities.

It was originally intended that HAZs would last for seven years. However, each new Secretary of State for Health appeared to bring a new focus for national health policy and, as a consequence, the potential future of HAZs became increasingly unclear. By 2000, the future funding available to HAZs had become less certain and the policy focus had shifted away from the original public health goals towards health service related issues. By 2002, a number of HAZs were being wound down. This made evaluating HAZs extremely difficult, particularly at national level for, even as the research teams collected data, the policy context and perceived aims of the HAZ programme were continually shifting. In addition, HAZs overlapped with similar area-based interventions, such as healthy living centres and local strategic partnerships. In some cases, this resulted in shared decision-making processes between different kinds of partnership, with HAZs "having no clear distinct and separate identity at local level" (Sullivan et al, 2002: 216). Hence, the ability for research to define precisely what the area-based initiatives labelled 'HAZs' had themselves achieved was restricted by the way in which the programme was conceived, rolled out and implemented. Overall, those in charge of the national evaluation concluded that key data employed in the national evaluation "do not support the view that HAZs made greater improvements to population health than non-HAZ areas between 1997 and 2001" (Bauld et al, 2005: 436) and that HAZs did not, therefore, substantially contribute to reducing health inequalities, as originally intended.

The Committee's report probably had little impact other than to keep the issue of public health and its importance alive within policy and media debates. It did, however, lead to one small tangible outcome, which was the publication of the final report of the CMO's Project to Strengthen the Public Health Function (Department of Health, 2001c). Despite being completed months earlier, it had not been published for reasons that had remained unclear. In the end, the report was published on the same day as the Health Committee's report in March 2001 (this review has already been commented on and is revisited in the sub-section below on workforce issues since 1997).

The next major policy development with implications for public health came when former banker, Derek Wanless, was commissioned by the then Chancellor of the Exchequer to examine future health trends and the resources required over a 20-year period (2002–22) to improve performance and deliver the *NHS Plan*. Unexpectedly, Wanless's report provided much-needed and welcome ammunition to those who had become concerned at the government's apparently weakening commitment to public health (Wanless, 2002). Wanless gave considerable prominence to public health and saw better measures in this area as essential to significantly reducing the growing demands for expensive health care interventions. He was critical of the current balance of care (and policy), which he argued focused too greatly on the acute hospital setting and inpatient beds. Improving the health of the public was portrayed as a means of 'investing in health', thereby lowering projected resource requirements for health care. Wanless did not say anything that those engaged with the public health function did not already know or had not sought to express on numerous occasions. Indeed, in its World Health Report 2002, the WHO reiterated its view that much scientific effort and most health resources were unwisely directed towards treating disease rather than preventing it (WHO, 2002). It called on governments to redress this imbalance, maintaining that it was a lack of political will that hindered progress. Nevertheless, the fact that Wanless was an outsider to these debates about public health and his background was rooted firmly in economics and the worlds of business and finance meant that his review marked an important development in post-1997 policy approaches to public health, paving the way for renewed interest in preventive approaches.

Underlying the Wanless review was a conviction that good health is good economics and that, far from being a cost, investment in health benefits the whole of society. What Wanless referred to as "the fully engaged scenario" (the other scenarios being "solid progress" and "low uptake" – see Box 4.3) involved a major shift in emphasis towards public health. The scenario assumed health would improve:

> dramatically with a sharp decline in key risk factors such as smoking and obesity, as people actively take ownership of their own health ... People have better diets and exercise much more ... These reductions in risk factors are assumed to be largest where they are currently highest, among people in the most deprived areas. This contributes to further reductions in socio-economic inequalities in health. (Wanless, 2002: 39)

Box 4.3: The Wanless scenarios

- **Slow uptake**: there is no change in the present level of public engagement; life expectancy rises by the lowest amount in all three scenarios and the health status of the population is constant or deteriorates. The health service is relatively unresponsive with low rates of technology uptake and low productivity.
- **Solid progress**: people become more engaged in relation to their health; life expectancy rises considerably, health status improves and people have confidence in the primary care system and use it more appropriately. The health service is responsive with high rates of technology and a more efficient use of resources.
- **Fully engaged**: levels of public engagement in relation to their health are high; life expectancy increases go beyond current forecasts, health status improves dramatically and people are confident in the health system and demand high quality care. The health service is responsive with high rates of technology uptake, particularly in relation to disease prevention. Use of resources is more efficient.

Source: Wanless (2004: 12)

In terms of addressing the issue of joined-up working across the NHS and local government in tackling health inequalities, Wanless argued that future health expenditure could only be reasonably contained by engaging the public in its health and reducing risky lifestyle behaviours (Wanless, 2002).

The government immediately signed up to the 'fully engaged scenario' and some short time later, in 2003, invited Wanless back to undertake a review of progress in meeting it. Although Wanless felt insufficient time had elapsed to say whether or not the government was on course to fulfil the scenario's requirements, he agreed to assess the direction of travel. However, this time he insisted his report should be addressed to the government and not merely to the Chancellor of the Exchequer. Consequently, he was able to ensure the Prime Minister and the Health Secretary (a post that had just been handed over from Alan Milburn to John Reid) both signed up to this second review and its terms of reference. Wanless's second report focused on the public health system as a whole and he produced a powerful critique of the public health function, which he argued lacked managerial grip, focus and capacity (Wanless, 2004). Perhaps not surprisingly, he found little had been achieved and recommended a range of changes, including an attempt to refocus the NHS from being an illness service to a health service. He was especially critical of PCTs, arguing that their small size made them ineffective in public health terms, and he considered the evidence base concerning why interventions succeeded or failed and how, if successful, they could be replicated more widely, was weak. However, he reserved his severest criticism for the failure of central government policy, noting that:

> Numerous policy statements and initiatives in the field of public health have not resulted in a rebalancing of policy away from health care ('a national sickness service') to health ('a national health service'). This will not happen until there is a realignment of incentives in the system to focus on reducing the burden of disease and tackling the key lifestyle and environmental risks. (Wanless, 2004: 23)

The government might have felt that such criticism was unfair or misplaced, as it had been engaged in a major initiative to strengthen partnerships in tackling health inequalities. Moreover, in 2003, the Department of Health had published *Tackling health inequalities: A programme for action*, which outlined how the findings of both the Treasury-led Cross-cutting Review of Tackling Health Inequalities (HM Treasury, 2002) and the Acheson Inquiry could be implemented. While the importance of mainstreamed and targeted activity was highlighted, this report made it clear that tackling health inequalities involved coordinating activity across traditional boundaries at governmental, regional and local levels, and working in partnership with "front-line staff, voluntary, community and business sectors as well as service users" (Department of Health, 2003a: 3). However, in his 2004 report, Wanless pointed out that the 'programme for action' gave no indication of costs or of how much various aspects of the strategy would contribute towards meeting the health inequalities targets, concluding that it would consequently be difficult to prioritise across the many possible interventions at a local level (Wanless, 2004: p 90, para 4.46).

The problem with policy approaches of the type favoured in the Department of Health's 'programme for action', which depend on partnership working, is that for the most part they are not being evaluated, so it is impossible to say how effective they are in influencing outcomes. Moreover, as we have seen, the structures themselves are subject to constant change and tinkering and therefore become insufficiently stable to allow partnerships to develop, mature and become sustainable (Perkins et al, 2010; Smith et al, 2009).

The government chose not to respond directly to Wanless's second report, preferring instead to focus on the production of a new health strategy to replace *Saving Lives*, published just five years earlier (Secretary of State for Health, 1999). Although the existing strategy still had to complete its course in terms of implementation, the government believed that there was now a need for a new and updated one, which would endeavour to do for public health what other strategies had done for the NHS in terms of modernisation. What this meant was a strategy replete with the vocabulary of health care reform that was by now familiar; there was a great deal of emphasis on personal choice and on providing information to people to enable them to make more informed decisions about their lifestyles. It was no longer considered acceptable, if it ever had been, for government to tell people how to lead their lives and risk being accused of acting as a 'nanny state'. As if to make this point as boldly as possible, the new strategy itself was informed by a major public consultation exercise in the lead-up to the final document and was given a title that overtly emphasised personal choice. *Choosing Health: Making Healthy Choices Easier* (Secretary of State for Health, 2004) marked a significant departure in terms of how the government saw its role in health improvement and tackling health inequalities. Whereas earlier statements had stressed the dual approach between government and individuals in promoting health, the new strategy shifted the focus far more firmly and explicitly towards the individual. The language around choice and individual responsibility in leading healthier lives was new, at least in a public health context, and the role of government was recast as an enabling, facilitating one designed to provide information and support to individuals who could use it to make healthier choices.

Similar language and objectives informed the health strategy published in 2006, *Our Health, Our Care, Our Say* (Secretary of State for Health, 2006). This White Paper came on the back of another round of major structural change in the NHS, which included halving the number of PCTs and modifying the roles of SHAs. An effort was also made to strengthen partnership working locally through the introduction of local area agreements from 2004/05. The strategy reiterated the government's commitment to health improvement and to better health outcomes. However, its influence was overshadowed by the organisational changes and financial problems sweeping across the NHS over this period. With fewer NHS organisations, job losses were inevitable and it took nearly two years to get the new structures in place and appoint senior managers to key posts. As with past NHS reorganisations, public health was not immune from such developments.

It was hardly surprising, therefore, that when Wanless came to undertake a more searching assessment of the government's attempts to implement his proposals for a 'fully engaged scenario', at the invitation of The King's Fund, he blamed the lack of progress on the constant reorganisation of the NHS and frequent policy initiatives, which had contributed little to the much needed improvements in health and instead served to divert management attention (Wanless et al, 2007). In particular, Wanless and his co-authors concluded that too little progress was being made with attempts to tackle complex public health challenges such as obesity and that, unless there was a major shift in direction, the fully engaged scenario to which the government had committed itself was unlikely to be realised. Indeed, as things stood, Wanless and colleagues argued that the government might not even achieve 'solid progress' and was instead somewhere between this and 'slow uptake' (see Box 4.3).

Two further, and final, policy milestones with implications for public health merit a mention. First is the NHS Next Stage Review, led by a surgeon turned junior health minister, Lord Darzi, which was undertaken in 2007 at the request of the incoming Prime Minister, Gordon Brown, with the aim of reconnecting clinicians with the reform agenda, placing them at the centre of future change. Darzi's final report was published in the summer of 2008 (Department of Health, 2008a). Although it mentions the importance of public health and the need for the NHS to work with local government, its focus is heavily on clinical care. Indeed, Darzi's review is a reassertion of the importance of quality of care and clinical governance – issues that New Labour had promoted during its initial years in office (Department of Health, 1998c). Moreover, much of the policy direction remains the same as that set out in the 2006 White Paper, *Our Health, Our Care, Our Say* (Secretary of State for Health, 2006). This direction was reinforced in Prime Minister Brown's first major speech on the NHS, delivered in January 2008, which placed a great deal of emphasis on secondary prevention and disease management (Brown, 2008). While there is obviously a public health dimension to these concerns and priorities, they form only part of the picture. As 2009 drew to a close, the public health system remained largely fragmented and appeared to have slipped down the government's policy agenda once again, although there were some countervailing pressures, notably the world class commissioning initiative (see later in this chapter) and related activities such as the joint strategic needs assessment (JSNA), and joint directors of public health appointments. It is too early to pass judgement on such developments, but in respect of JSNA a review of progress so far, which has been conducted by the Improvement and Development Agency (IDeA), concludes that "the signs are good" and that "the JSNA story so far is looking positive" (Hughes, 2009: 21). Nevertheless, the challenge remains one of how positive processes in respect of establishing joint priorities and effective partnerships can be translated into actions that have real impact on outcomes for people. Much the same applies to joint DsPH posts, which have been the subject of another IDeA review (Hunter (ed), 2008). The principle of joint posts has been widely welcomed, but much unfinished business remains to ensure that they are both viable and effective when it comes to meeting public health objectives. So far, such posts have lacked independent and systematic study. In his critical appraisal of them, Elson (2008) emphasises the need for more transparency about how the post is to be used and argues that remits ought to be matched to the needs of the local context.

All may not be lost on the wider policy front either. A reminder of the importance of the wider public health system came in August 2008 in the form of the report of the WHO Commission on Social Determinants of Health (WHO, 2008a). Adopting a social justice perspective, the authors concluded that: "action on the social determinants of health must involve the whole of government, civil society and local communities, business, global fora, and international agencies. Policies and programmes must embrace all the key sectors of society not just the health sector" (WHO, 2008a: 1). Health ministries were called on to "champion a social determinants of health approach" and "support other ministries in creating policies that promote health equity". Responsibility for the health gap was attributed to a "toxic combination of bad policies, economics, and politics" (WHO, 2008a: 26) and the following three principles of action were advocated:

- improve the conditions of daily life – the circumstances in which people are born, grow, live, work and age;

- tackle the inequitable distribution of power, money, and resources – and the structural drivers of those conditions of daily life – globally, nationally and locally;
- measure the problem, evaluate action, expand the knowledge base, develop a workforce that is trained in the social determinants of health and raise public awareness about the social determinants of health.

In reviewing its own approach to tackling health inequalities in England, and in order to learn the lessons from the WHO Commission, apply them locally and identify what else needed to be done, the government, at the end of 2008, set up a commission chaired by Michael Marmot, which reported to the Health Secretary at the end of 2009 (Marmot also chaired the WHO's global Commission on the Social Determinants of Health). The review was established with the aim of proposing an evidence-based strategy for reducing health inequalities from 2010 (see Box 4.4).

Box 4.4: Marmot review's tasks

- Identify the evidence most relevant to underpinning future policy and action to meet the health inequalities challenge facing England.
- Show how this evidence could be translated into practice.
- Advise on possible objectives and measures, building on the experience of the current public service agreement (PSA) target on infant mortality and life expectancy.
- Publish a report of the review's work, which will contribute to the development of a post-2010 health inequalities strategy.

A principal concern of the review was to examine the levers and incentives to ensure effective implementation of policy and bring about change, including interagency working, (economic and other) incentives, the role of targets and indicators, and workforce implications.

In its final report, the review concluded that national policies would fail to reduce inequalities if local delivery systems were unable to deliver them (Marmot Review, 2010). It accepted the evidence received from local practitioners that they wanted freedom to develop locally appropriate plans to reduce health inequalities within nationally agreed principles. The review proposed that strategic policy should be underpinned by a limited number of aspirational targets that supported the intended strategic direction to impove and reduce disparities in life and health expectancy and monitor child development and social inclusion across the social gradient. The role of local government was seen to be pivotal both to improve health and to reduce health inequalities. Although the need for strong partnerships between local authorities and NHS PCTs was stressed, it was acknowledged that the current partnership framework needed considerable development and enhancement with less focus on targets, which often reinforced silo-working, and more attention to a whole systems perspective. Appropriate leadership skills were also needed and should be invested in to ensure that partnerships were effective.

Setting targets and performance managing

Another important departure in the post-1997 Labour government's approach to health has been a focus on targets and performance assessment. This focus has been extended to health improvement and health inequalities, for which targets have also been set, although arguably without the same degree of commitment or consistency as applied to others, particularly access targets (Hunter and Marks, 2005; Marks and Hunter, 2005). For example, the 1999 health strategy *Saving Lives: Our Healthier Nation* set out various health improvement targets in particular 'health problem areas', such as coronary heart disease and cancer. Since then, a series of changes and additions to targets of relevance to public health have been made, including the introduction of health inequalities targets focusing on life expectancy and infant mortality (Department of Health, 2001a) as well as targets focusing on changing lifestyle behaviours, such as smoking. Public health was one of the seven domains for which core and developmental standards were monitored by the Healthcare Commission as part of its Annual Health Check (Healthcare Commission, 2004). The Healthcare Commission was replaced by the Care Quality Commission in April 2009. At the time of writing, its approach to monitoring and inspection is undergoing changes to publish more timely data, although it is likely to retain much of its predecessor's approach and method. This includes assessments of conformity with public health guidance from NICE and developmental standards that emphasise the importance of a whole systems approach. In addition to the notion that targets should act as drivers for action, some of the broader public service agreement targets were used to promote collaboration between local government and the NHS through shared responsibility for outcomes and have since been absorbed into local area agreements (LAAs), agreed across central government and a local area, and across the partnerships within local areas. From April 2009, LAAs were assessed through a comprehensive area assessment (CAA) led by the Audit Commission (Audit Commission et al, 2009). The CAA replaced the comprehensive performance assessment of local government and makes all partners within a local authority area, including PCTs, accountable for shared outcomes.

Developments in the workforce: making a reality of multidisciplinary public health

Perhaps as a consequence of the lack of a clear conception of its purpose and raison d'être, the public health function has been subjected to a considerable degree of change and uncertainty. As was asserted in a recent House of Lords debate: "Nowhere, perhaps, has reorganisation been more disruptive than in public health" (House of Lords, 2006). For ease of reference, and to avoid cluttering the main text with the numerous structural changes that have occurred with increasing rapidity since 1974, the various changes are described in the Appendix. As noted earlier, these changes have invariably not been directed primarily at the public health community but have nevertheless had a major impact on policy and practice at all levels of the system. This is particularly true of those sections of the workforce employed by, or working for, the NHS. All these developments have resulted in a public health community that is increasingly insecure and unsure of its purpose or fitness for whatever that purpose proves to be. This was borne out by the comments made by many of our interviewees, some of whom testified to the resulting poor morale within the public health community:

> PCT: I've seen lots of colleagues who have just said this is enough, and honestly I'm feeling I couldn't cope with … getting my head around yet another reorganisation … So I think it's really tough keeping morale up now.

> NGO: None of the money that's promised for public health has seen itself through … I mean it's an absolute scandal. Yes, people are leaving the profession, the cuts are big … have been throughout the system. Morale is very, very low indeed. And also they're worn out with organisational change.

Despite the constant policy and organisational churn in evidence from 1997 to the present, there were also some encouraging developments for the public health workforce, particularly with respect to strengthening its multidisciplinary base. Soon after the government had entered office, there followed a detailed commitment to developing multidisciplinary public health, including a specific pledge to creating a new, non-medical role of specialist in public health in the White Paper, *Saving Lives: Our Healthier Nation* (Secretary of State for Health, 1999). This announced a number of initiatives intended to help develop a genuinely multidisciplinary public health function. These included the production of a National Public Health Workforce Development Plan (which, although virtually completed, was never published), the completion of a Public Health Skills Audit, the creation of a Public Health Development Fund and the establishment of the post of specialist in public health, which, it claimed, would "be of equivalent status in independent practice to medically qualified consultants in public health medicine and allow [non-clinical public health specialists] to become directors of public health" (Secretary of State for Health, 1999: 136). The same White Paper also announced the establishment of the Health Development Agency (replacing the Health Education Authority), which was charged with a mandate to build and disseminate the evidence base for public health and to facilitate the sharing of knowledge and good practice.

The following year Alan Milburn, then Secretary of State for Health, gave the London School of Economics and Political Science annual health lecture, in which he called on those involved in public health to end "lazy thinking and occupational protectionism" and "take public health out of the ghetto" (Milburn, 2000):

> [T]he time has come to take public health out of the ghetto. For too long the overarching label 'public health' has served to bundle together functions and occupations in a way that actually marginalizes them. So by a series of definitional sleights of hand the argument runs that the health of the population should be mainly improved by population-level health promotion and prevention, which in turn is best delivered – or at least overseen and managed – by medical consultants in public health. The time has come to abandon this lazy thinking and occupational protectionism.

In 2000, the year after the first consultant-level specialist public health posts to be open to candidates from disciplines other than medicine were advertised by some health authorities, the Faculty of Public Health Medicine agreed that membership of the Faculty should be opened to candidates from disciplines other than medicine and dropped 'Medicine' from its title, becoming the Faculty of Public Health. Also in 2001, as mentioned in earlier chapters, the final *Report of the Chief Medical Officer's Project to Strengthen the Public Health Function* was published (Department of Health, 2001c), providing further support for the earlier policy statements' calls for a multidisciplinary approach to public health. This report identified three broad categories of people comprising the public health workforce:

- **Specialists**: consultants in public health medicine and specialists in public health who work at a strategic or senior management level or at a senior level of scientific expertise to influence the health of the population or of a selected community.
- **Public health practitioners**: those who spend a major part, or all, of their time in public health practice – for example, health visitors and school nurses.
- **Wider public health**: most people, including managers, who have a role in health improvement and reducing health inequalities although they may not recognise this, including teachers, social workers, local business leaders, transport engineers, town planners, housing officers, regeneration managers and so on.

This categorisation, which does not suggest medical training is essential for individuals working in any of the three categories, remains central to Department of Health policy. The CMO's report also highlighted problems of undercapacity in the public health workforce and recommended significant government action to address the deficit:

> We need to make sure that the public health workforce across all sectors is skilled, staffed, and resourced to deal with the major task of delivering the Government's health strategy. An increase in capacity and capabilities must be achieved. (Department of Health, 2001c: 24)

Importantly, the report suggests that a renewed drive to increase public health workforce capacity should be accompanied by moves to ensure the workforce becomes more multidisciplinary in nature. However, identifying exactly who or what comprises the public health workforce has created problems. Crowley and Hunter (2005: 265), for instance, argue that:

> ... greater clarity and focus is required if public health is to deliver ... especially in respect of health improvement that

demands skills from a range of agencies outside the NHS and located within communities.

A number of studies have assessed the impact of the 2002 NHS reorganisation on public health. For example, one study found that medically qualified specialists were less skilled in community development, leadership and management (Barts and City University London, 2003). Gaps in information analysis skills were common. Another study of the capacity and capabilities of the public health workforce found there was:

- a lack of clarity surrounding the term 'specialist in public health' and confusion regarding both the role of a specialist and the general public health function;
- fragmentation of the workforce;
- a loss of critical mass and the potential for professional isolation; key skills gaps including health protection, partnership working and leadership (Chapman, Shaw et al, 2005).

Between 2001 and 2002, the Faculty of Public Health gradually opened up its public health examinations to non-medical candidates. Within the new PCTs, of which there were over 300 arising from *Shifting the Balance of Power* (Department of Health, 2001d), the first directors of public health from backgrounds other than medicine were appointed, and the Minister for Public Health at the time officially welcomed the fact that "this generation of DsPH come from a variety of backgrounds – both medical and non-medical" (Blears, 2002). She also welcomed the new DsPH who were jointly appointed by both the NHS and local government, suggesting that such developments provided cause for optimism "that multidisciplinary public health will become a reality" (Blears, 2002). However, to allay any fears about substitution or marginalisation, she also stressed that doctors "remain a crucial part of this new world" (Blears, 2002). Also at this time, and in keeping with the renewed emphasis on strengthening the wider public health workforce, the UK Voluntary Register for Public Health Specialists was established in 2003 to help quality assure this new breed of non-clinical specialists; the first trainee from a background other than medicine successfully completed their training through the Faculty of Public Health route in 2005, by which time one third of the Faculty's 3,000+ members were from backgrounds other than medicine (Evans and Knight, 2006).

Many of those involved in public health have welcomed the expansion of public health responsibilities to include a wider range of players (for example, Wright, 2007). However, the shift away from a requirement for public health specialists to have medical training towards a more inclusive approach has not been without opposition, as a series of debates in the *British Medical Journal* in 2000/01 illustrates (for example, McPherson, 2000; McPherson et al, 2001). Wright (2007: 219) claims that medical resistance focused on concerns about whether the route to such specialist posts open to non-medical specialists (achieved via a portfolio approach) constituted real equivalence to the route taken by medically qualified personnel, suggesting it was perhaps "an easy alternative to higher specialist training".

There were also concerns that public health might lose its critical mass, with Jessop (2002: 1) warning: "NHS public health workers will be dispersed to the loneliness of 300 primary care trusts ... they will face professional isolation, with hence an inevitable struggle to retain competence and sanity". To counter the fragmentation of the public health workforce, the government announced the establishment of public health networks (Department of Health, 2001d) – see Box 4.5.

Box 4.5: Public health networks

As Mallinson and colleagues point out,

> ... it is important to distinguish Public Health Networks ... from other forms of self-defining and regulating networks ... [S]ince the establishment of PHNs was part of a centrally steered restructuring of health services, they are different from many of the networks described in ... academic literatures. This was, in part, why they were originally mooted as 'managed' networks. (Mallinson et al, 2006: 261)

In practice, central government has provided very little steer as to how public health networks ought to be structured, leaving their formation up to local decision makers. As might be expected in such circumstances, a variety of different types of public health network have subsequently emerged (Fahey et al, 2003). For example, Abbott and Killoran (2005) identify networks operating at four different levels of NHS organisation, with varying memberships and contrasting conceptualisations as to what the purpose and objectives of the networks are. Hence, in considering the role that such networks might play in countering fragmentation, there is a need first to clarify what is meant by the term 'public health network'. Without this clarity, Fahey and colleagues note:

... when a speaker/writer uses this term [public health network] the audience are often unsure if they are referring to a specific type of public health network, the government definition of a network, the faculty definition, or some all encompassing term. (Fahey et al, 2003: 938)

There are some similarities between the various definitions of public health networks, which seem largely to aspire to help pool expertise and skills in specialist areas of public health, provide a means of sharing good practice, manage public health knowledge, and act as a source of learning and professional development. However, as Fahey and colleagues (2003) highlight, there are also key differences. For example, in the Faculty of Public Health's (2007) definition, public health networks are expected to play a role in public accountability and in ensuring programmes can be performance managed, whereas *Shifting the Balance of Power* (Department of Health, 2001d) explicitly states that public health networks are not linked to performance management regimes.

It is perhaps unsurprising therefore that, in a survey of 60 public health professionals working in England, Fahey and colleagues (2003) found that understandings of the term 'public health network' varied considerably from person to person and, overall, that their definitions tended to be somewhat broader than the government's. This research led Fahey and colleagues to construct their own definition of a public health network as:

A network of public health professionals within a defined geographic area which facilitates communication, information sharing and linking of those with common interests/skills to enable efficient working across organisational boundaries to deliver the public health function. (Fahey et al, 2003: 941)

More recently, a postal questionnaire survey of a random sample of members and fellows of the Faculty of Public Health by other researchers (Connelly et al, 2005) supports the idea that there remains no clear consensus about what a public health network is, even among public health professionals. Their results found that 69% of the 229 respondents reported feeling that 'public health networks' were inadequately defined, with the majority also suggesting that public health networks are underdeveloped and lack coordination, purpose and structure. What seems clear from these findings is that public health networks have tended to focus on links between various public health *specialists,* so it is unclear to what extent, if at all, this has progressed the multidisciplinary nature of the public health workforce (Abbott et al, 2005). In the light of this finding, some researchers (for example, Mallinson et al, 2006) have criticised the trajectory of the development of public health networks to date for favouring a traditional public health function and membership.

There are also concerns about the extent to which the moves towards a multidisciplinary workforce have actually succeeded. As Wright (2007: 219) points out, the new route for non-medical specialists was, in reality, open to relatively few senior professionals, "leaving a disaffected and unsupported majority of the workforce in need of further training" to reach the levels of competence required. In 2001, the House of Commons Health Committee (2001) claimed that the government had failed to redress the balance between health care and health. A year later, Evans and Dowling (2002) reported that significant barriers to multidisciplinary public health persist, including a continuing lack of clarity about policy aims combined with a belief that training, registration and career pathways remain unclear for individuals who do not have medical qualifications. In 2003, Evans wrote:

> Despite the rhetoric of inclusion and equivalence, in practice there is continuing demarcation between medical and non-medical public health jobs. Regional director of public health posts and consultants in communicable disease control remain restricted to medical candidates. Non-medical directors of public health in PCTs earn between £15–20,000 less than medical colleagues apparently doing the same jobs. Although the FPHM [Faculty of Public Health Medicine] has opened its examinations and membership to non-medical candidates on an equivalent basis, there are many structures that remain essentially uni-disciplinary. (Evans, 2003: 965)

Closely related to the tensions between medical expertise and the drive for a multidisciplinary workforce, long-standing debates about the best location for the public health function have remained alive (Hunter, 2003). The retention of the major public health function within the NHS is linked to the survival of the speciality of public health medicine and yet, as Hunter (2003: 111) claims: "All available evidence suggests that the NHS, essentially a 'sickness' service, will never take the wider public health seriously". The belief that it is irrational to maintain the location of the majority of public health specialists within the NHS when most of the major levers for achieving public health's aims lie beyond the NHS is supported by the evidence that the first joint Director of Public Health to be appointed in England, Dr Andrew Richards, presented to the House of Commons Health Committee's inquiry into public health in 2001 in a memorandum (House of Commons Health Committee, 2001b: 442). He argued that "the location of DsPH at the heart of the NHS has inevitably pulled them away from, rather than towards, those parts of the wider system that most powerfully influence health". In support of joint DsPH appointments, he considered it to be "irrational that most of the interest, skills and resources to improve public health are outside the NHS while the DPH is locked into it". Therefore, "there are strong arguments that DsPH have to be eased out of the NHS box".

The Labour government's second White Paper on public health, *Choosing Health: Making Healthier Choices Easier* (Secretary of State for Health, 2004), demonstrates how important it is for those working in public health to look beyond the NHS. It highlights six key themes for public health, all of which require engagement by partners beyond the NHS – notably, local government but also other agencies – sexual health, mental health, tackling obesity, smoking reduction, reduction in alcohol intake and reduction generally in health inequalities. The crucial role of the public health workforce is emphasised with regards to achieving the desired behavioural changes in all of these areas. Annex B of *Choosing Health* considers the importance of ensuring public health practitioners have the correct skills for their work in improving health, including a strong leadership capacity, and makes commitments to addressing critical shortfalls in specific staff groups.

Given Wanless's criticisms about the weak implementation of public health policy, the issue of delivery was a key one for the architects of the public health White Paper. An accompanying document, which was published some months later, *Delivering Choosing Health* (Department of Health, 2005a), outlines the government's commitment to developing the public health workforce as a key means of improving health and tackling health inequalities. In the Supporting Strategy B of this document (pp 42-3), it is suggested that new contractual arrangements within the NHS ought to be used to engage primary care staff in improving health through everyday practice. This section also outlines the development of some new roles within the field of public health, including health trainers, which were proposed in the *Choosing Health* White Paper. Health trainers were to be recruited from local communities and were funded to offer tailored information, motivation and practical support to individuals and groups who were interested in adopting healthier lifestyles, helping them to set personal goals in areas such as stopping smoking, doing more exercise, eating healthy foods, practising safe sex, dealing with stress and tackling social isolation. They were also intended to identify barriers to healthier choices and signpost people to relevant local services. The initiative has been described as "taking the NHS to people" (Secretary of State for Health, 2004).

As well as encouraging local delivery and strategic plans to help identify gaps in the workforce, the delivery plan suggests a national workforce strategy and competency framework is required "to underpin the development of education, skills and work across the health and social care community, local government, business communities and the voluntary sector" (Department of Health, 2005a: 42). A single public health skills and career framework was subsequently produced, having been developed in response to an expressed need for a mechanism that "facilitates collaboration and coherence across this diverse workforce" (Public Health Resource Unit and Skills for Health, 2008: 4). The framework is designed to help "ensure rigour and consistency in skills, competence and knowledge at all levels, regardless of professional background, and by enabling flexible public health career progression" (Public Health Resource Unit and Skills for Health, 2008: 4). For the first time, it brings together into one development framework the various standards, competencies and training routes pursued separately by each professional group.

Another important development has been a desire to achieve some degree of role and pay parity between public health practitioners with clinical and non-clinical backgrounds. A government initiative entitled *Agenda for Change* (Department of Health, 2004) aimed to bring the whole of the NHS workforce (with the exception of doctors and dentists) into a single pay framework. Although this policy was not specifically intended to unify the public health workforce, Wright (2007) argues that the changes it has brought about are leading to a coherent approach to job definitions and pay scales in public health for the first time. The absence of alignment has been a major stumbling block in terms of encouraging non-clinicians to enter the public health workforce.

A subsequent White Paper, *Our Health, Our Care, Our Say* (Secretary of State for Health, 2006), placed further emphasis on the need to develop the capacity of, and skills within, the health workforce. It pointed out that, currently, very little of the money the NHS and social care sectors spend on training goes on training people in support roles and argues that "it is not acceptable that some of the most dependent people in our communities are cared for by the least well trained" (Secretary of State for Health, 2006: 188). The document goes on to make commitments to spending more money on training and support for the wider health and care workforce, and to developing joint service and workforce planning between the NHS and local authorities. It is not yet clear what progress, if any, has been made in achieving these aims.

Alongside these developments, important changes among the various NGOs and professional groups involved in public health have occurred over the last decade (see Box 4.6).

Box 4.6: NGOs and the public health workforce

It is generally accepted that NGOs, including voluntary organisations and community groups, have had a significant part to play in the development of public health and that their potential to engage in healthy public policy decision making should be encouraged (Scriven, 2007b). Much of their work impacts on the public health workforce in a variety of ways, from devising and accrediting competencies and skill sets to lobbying for changes in policy and practice. However, the precise role of NGOs in influencing policy or helping to shape the climate of public opinion over a public health issue is less easy to discern and does not appear to be well documented. In one of the witness seminars exploring the evolution of public health since the 1970s, the contribution of NGOs was specifically mentioned by one of the witnesses who singled out:

> ... the big campaign groups who were identifying the health consequences of environmental issues, such as Greenpeace, Friends of the Earth. There was also a group I joined called 'British Scientists for Social Responsibility', I don't suppose that one's still going! But these were having an effect, not just in forming popularist opinion but in terms of influence, for example, on the Royal Commission on Environmental Pollution that actually brought about law on all kinds of things. (Evans and Knight, 2006: 12)

Despite this kind of anecdotal evidence, however, documented examples of where NGOs have made a particular contribution to public health policy decisions are not plentiful, although this could be a consequence of the rather mysterious and opaque nature of policy making in the UK (see Burton, 2001). Indeed, few would dispute that such bodies remain an important sector within the public health system and clearly contribute in respect of highlighting problems, generating new thinking, providing a platform for those with particular expertise and serving as channels for lobbying and advocacy efforts.

NGOs comprise international bodies like WHO; national public health bodies advocating for improved health, such as the UK Public Health Association (UKPHA); national bodies set up by, but independent from, government that are concerned with aspects of public health, such as the Food Standards Agency; and campaigning bodies that focus on particular public health topics or issues, such as the National Heart Forum, National Obesity Forum, Alcohol Concern and Action on Smoking and Health (ASH).

The launch of the UKPHA in 1999 signified an important development for public health as it brought together three pre-existing organisations: the Public Health Alliance, the Association for Public Health and the Public Health Trust (which was the charitable arm of the Public Health Alliance). Its aim was to unite the public health movement in the UK. Unfortunately, despite several initiatives, such unification has proved more difficult to achieve than expected, although perhaps this should come as no surprise given the failed attempts of earlier initiatives to bring together various public health organisations. However, the issue has once again risen up the agenda with a former Minister for Public Health, Caroline Flint, voicing concerns about fragmentation within the public health community and the number of bodies claiming to speak on behalf of public health. As a consequence, fresh moves are under way to see, once again, if there is scope to integrate further key public health bodies, namely, the Faculty of Public Health, Royal Institute of Public Health (RIPH), Royal Society for the Promotion of Health (RSH), UK Public Health Association, and the Chartered Institute of Environmental Health Officers. As part of this rationalisation, in June 2007, the RIPH and RSH announced their intention to merge. The so-called 'royal wedding' took place on 1 October 2008 and the new merged body is known as the Royal Society for Public Health (RSPH). However, with the RSPH in place and the Faculty of Public Health having successfully sought member support to seek separate Royal College status (rather than being part of the Royal College of Physicians), the likelihood of greater unity among public health NGOs seems small in the foreseeable future. A limited move in this direction is the likely merger of the UKPHA's annual public health forum with the Faculty's annual conference. The first such joint conference is scheduled for 2011.

In addition, attempts have been made to encourage primary care professionals to focus more explicitly on preventative health measures. For example, the new GP contract, implemented in 2004, allows for payment to be tailored to specific services and was partially intended to develop further the health promotion aspects of this key primary care function. However, as Peckham and Exworthy (2003) note, primary care in the UK has been primarily focused on general practice working within a medical model of health. The social model on which public health draws has generally been the exception in primary care. In her evidence to the Health Committee's inquiry into public health, Professor Jennie Popay referred to the "awesome" expectations laid on primary care to deliver the public health agenda, noting the absence of evidence to suggest that GPs either "have the capacity or the inclination" to move upstream (House of Commons Health Committee, 2001b: 91).

How far have things changed?

Despite the promising policy rhetoric around public health, the structural reorganisation of the public health function, and commitment to developing public health practitioners and the specialist workforce, the recent literature on the public health workforce makes for disappointing reading and does not suggest that the problems outlined by Brackenridge (1981) and others over 20 years ago have yet been fully dealt with. Time after time, more recent research on a range of different sectors and aspects of the public health workforce has cited problems of undercapacity and a lack of clarity around training, career progression and interdisciplinary working. For example, Brown's (2002) scoping study of the public health workforce in the North East, Yorkshire and Humber found a great deal of consensus among members that it was under capacity, under resourced, had skill gaps and that there were significant organisational difficulties in promoting collaborative and integrated working. The findings from this study (which are discussed further in Brown and Learmonth, 2005) also indicate that problems around professional barriers and 'turf wars' were impeding partnership working, and that there had been little practical progress in terms of building capacity across the three levels of the workforce identified by the CMO (Department of Health, 2001c; see also above) because of a lack of resources.

Studies on the role of public health nurses have found problems in training and associated gaps in skills, a lack of clarity of individuals' roles and experiences of marginalisation from other members of the public health and healthcare workforces (Burke et al, 2001; Latter et al, 2003). Research on the role of public health specialists (for example, Chapman, Abbott et al, 2005; Chapman, Shaw et al, 2005; Gray et al, 2005) identifies key skills gaps, a lack of clarity over the role of the specialist and the public health function, fragmentation and attrition of the workforce, and inadequacies in training and continuing professional development.

Around the same time as these various critical accounts emerged, a report commissioned jointly by the Department of Health and the Welsh Assembly Government (2004), which aimed to tackle some of these issues, was published. Acknowledging many of the problems outlined above, the report sought to help define the roles, functions and development needs of the specialist public health workforce. In the context of the White Paper *Choosing Health* (Secretary of State for Health, 2004), this report focuses particularly on the health promotion aspect of public health specialists' roles. It recommends long-term sustainable staffing structures (and associated funding), a clear and recognised career pathway allowing free movement between the NHS and local government, and supporting education and training.

The prospects for better public health education and training may be constrained, however, as evidence suggests that the academic side of public health is also struggling with a range of difficulties. An investigation into academic public health raised serious concerns about capacity and identified significant problems with the funding of academic posts (Public Health Sciences Working Group, 2004):

> The report highlights the extraordinary disparity between, on the one hand, the overriding importance of the public health sciences for public protection, service provision and health improvement and, on the other, the limited strategic interest that is taken in their infrastructure and conduct. Impressive achievements in the biomedical sciences and medical care can obscure the fact that the circumstances in which people live, whether these circumstances are under their personal control or not, are still the major determinants of health. (Public Health Sciences Working Group, 2004: 2)

Consecutive surveys of the specialist public health workforce, undertaken by the Faculty of Public Health in 2003 and 2005, also highlight issues of undercapacity in the specialist section of the public health workforce (Gray et al, 2005; Gray and Sandberg, 2006). These surveys indicate that there was a fall in numbers of consultants/specialists in public health of 17% (224 individuals) in the UK between 2003 and 2005, reducing the overall level of total specialist public health capacity in the UK from 22.2 per million in 2003 to 18.5 per million in 2005 (Gray and Sandberg, 2006). The report's authors claim that this fall appears to have related particularly to public health specialists working in the NHS in England and in universities. In addition, the surveys found evidence of significant regional variation in the distribution of public health specialists, widespread dissatisfaction with public health team capacity and a significant proportion of specialists (17.6%) who were considering leaving the speciality within the next five years.

Problems with undercapacity in the public health workforce are noted by the CMO in his 2005 annual report (Department of Health, 2006), which highlights a deficit in public health capacity affecting the 48% of England's population living in the Midlands and the North. The report also suggests public health funds are being "raided" to support clinical activities in some areas. In light of this, the CMO suggests that the lack of progress "is more compatible with the Wanless 'slow uptake' scenario than with the 'fully engaged' scenario" to which the government is ostensibly committed (Department of Health, 2006: 39). In conclusion, the CMO suggests consideration should be given to "establishing a comprehensive review (the first in almost 20 years) into arrangements to improve and safeguard the health of the public" (Department of Health, 2006: 45).

While such a review seems unlikely, other developments have occurred. For example, following the recommendation of *Delivering Choosing Health* (Department of Health, 2005a) that a national workforce and competency framework was required, plans to develop a coherent public health career framework for use across the UK have been implemented. As mentioned earlier, this work, which was undertaken by Skills for Health and the Public Health Resource Unit (on behalf of the Department of Health), has sought to create a simple and easy-to-use tool to facilitate collaboration and coherence across the diverse public health workforce.

The framework, which is aimed at the development not only of the professional public health workforce but also the wider workforce, is based on a modified version of the generic NHS Career Framework. It consists of nine levels, from initial entry to the public health system to the most senior positions in relevant organisations. Each level contains descriptions of the main competencies and knowledge required to work at that level. Public health work is based on various competencies, in a combination of core areas, which everyone in the field is expected to have, and non-core areas, which apply to more specific domains of public health. These competencies relate closely to the ten areas of public health practice that underpin the UK Voluntary Register for Public Health Specialists. The revised competencies already form the basis for the job description of directors of public health (Faculty of Public Health, 2006).

The core areas are:

- surveillance and assessment of the population's health and wellbeing;
- assessing the evidence of effectiveness of interventions, programmes and services to improve population health and wellbeing;

- policy and strategy development and implementation for population health and wellbeing;
- leadership and collaborative working for population health and wellbeing.

The non–core areas are:

- health improvement;
- health protection;
- public health intelligence;
- academic public health;
- health and social care quality.

Following testing of the framework, necessary changes have been made to ensure that it is fit for purpose, although it will continue to evolve as the workforce and the focus of public health policy change. This will be especially important in the context of recent changes in public services, notably the NHS and local government. These include a greater emphasis on commissioning and on making a clear distinction between this and the provision of services, better partnership working, and more diversity of service providers with a bigger role envisaged for new third sector social enterprises. In addition, further work is required in respect of public health leadership development, including reaching an agreement as to what further work might be undertaken in this area to provide appropriate leadership programmes for director-level staff. Some progress has been made in this area with the Improvement Foundation working with Durham University and the local government IDeA to offer a new national Leading Improvement for Health and Well-being Programme (Hannaway et al, 2007). In addition, the NHS North West has also launched an Aspiring Directors of Public Health Leadership Programme being run by the consultancy group Salomon's.

How is progress viewed on the ground?

Our interviewees were asked whether they considered the public health workforce to be multidisciplinary and to discuss which skills they felt were required by this workforce. Opinions about the extent to which the current public health workforce (at the time of the interviews) was multidisciplinary depended on the way in which they defined 'multidisciplinary'. Those who suggested a multidisciplinary workforce already existed either felt that not everyone who contributed to it necessarily saw public health as part of their role (and that this was relatively unimportant), or had a rather narrow view of what constituted a multidisciplinary workforce. For example, the following interviewee fell into the former category:

> DH: I often have to pinch myself before I get into a debate about the public health workforce because I don't actually think of this group of people with sort of public health workforce labels and t-shirts on as they go round. I think of people across the whole of the public sector who have some aspects of public health work within their role and remit and who make a contribution. And therefore I don't actually necessarily usually distinguish between a group of full-time public health professionals and the broader public health or health improvement role of people who work in Housing or Education or in Benefits Services or in the NHS, in fact. So I always struggle when we get into this debate and I think that sometimes we almost create a bit of a paper tiger.

In contrast, the following interviewee presented a rather narrower view of 'multidisciplinary', defining it merely in terms of the mix of medical and non-medical specialists:

> PCT: [A multidisciplinary workforce] is very much a reality, certainly here … I'm intending that, when my consultant posts are all filled, they should be a mix of medical and non-medical posts. In pure numbers' terms, the majority of people who work in the public health directorate are non-medical.

Indeed, the divide between interviewees who focused on a medical model of health and those who focused on wider social and economic determinants was quite stark in several aspects of the data but particularly in relation to discussions about the workforce. For example, the following two interviewees were both keen to emphasise that they felt medical expertise was essential to achieving public health objectives, or at least to undertaking certain aspects of the work that are currently expected of DsPH. In this regard, it is important to distinguish between belief in a medical model of health on the one hand and recognition of the tasks that fall to DsPH in PCTs on the other (one of which is control of health care associated infections):

> PCT: I think that it would be a disaster if we don't maintain a fair number of medics in public health because I do think that medics have got a particular contribution to make.

> PCT [different interviewee from above]: I'm conscious of what I do, in my day-to-day job, a huge amount of it is not technically public health. I'm a Medical Director but also I cover a huge number of other things because I have a clinical background and because I'm jolly experienced at this, that and the other.

However, many other interviewees, especially those based in local and central government and in NGOs, felt that the dominance of a model of public health in which medical professionals were accorded higher status than non-medical professionals was a major cause of many of the problems dogging the current public health system. In fact, an interviewee based at the Department of Health (DH) expressed frustration that some public health specialists working within central government did not take his/her views seriously because s/he did not have medical training:

> DH: I'm reflecting some of my own frustrations around trying to get my colleagues in public health to take anything that I do in this area seriously because I'm not a doctor. I've found it very easy to get a lot of other people to change but I've found it enormously difficult ... It's funny, isn't it? You know, here I am [in the Department of Health in a public health role] and the people I've had most difficulty getting any engagement with in national policy are the people running public health.

While, on the whole, those subscribing to a narrow definition of the public health workforce tended to be public health specialists who had undertaken medical training and those who emphasised the importance of a model of public health that focused on wider determinants of health tended to have non-medical backgrounds, this was not consistently the case. It is important to emphasise that many public health specialists (DsPH and RDsPH) were extremely supportive of the need to include a broad and diverse mix of skills in the public health workforce and were generally encouraging about the potential for people from outside the traditional public health community to move into public health specialist posts. Furthermore, the majority of interviewees felt that progress had been made over the last five years, despite professional resistance from some 'old-fashioned public health leaders', and this was perceived to be embodied in the increasing number of joint appointments and teams straddling the NHS and local authorities. Nevertheless, with the exception of the few interviewees who felt that a multidisciplinary workforce already existed, most of the interviewees suggested this was an area that still required a great deal of further development.

This suggests that efforts over recent years to encourage the specialist public health workforce to broaden its constituency, and to link more closely with actors and sectors beyond the specialist workforce, are having an impact, although it is hard to judge precisely what this might be in the absence of systematic evidence. While it is true that mechanisms such as local strategic partnerships and local area agreements have been widely welcomed, the evidence concerning their impact on outcomes is hard to come by (Perkins et al, 2010). Bearing in mind that the shift in outlook on the part of public health specialists requires cultural as well as policy change and that it is dependent on a range of factors, including changes in training programmes, it is unsurprising that this shift has not occurred quickly.

A significant number of interviewees reported that recruitment to public health specialist posts remained problematic and expressed a range of concerns, including the limited resources available to public health and the difficulties caused by the raft of recent reforms (both issues have already been touched on and are discussed further in Chapter Five). As a consequence, several of the interviewees felt that there was a worrying dissonance between the skills required by new specialist public health posts and those that were being promoted through the various career routes to these posts. For example:

> SHA: We've got this problem that the new public health directors require a new set of skills, and I don't think that public health was really prepared for that, and I think over the last five years we've failed to train people with the right skills to deliver on the new agenda. And it's been really hard to recruit high quality directors of public health – we just can't find them.

The skills that were mentioned most often as those that public health training courses failed to address but that candidates for specialist posts were expected to possess related to: commissioning, collaborative working, leadership and financial management (key themes that are all discussed further in Chapter Five). Unfortunately, while most interviewees felt this was an area that ought to be addressed, few of the interviewees working within the specialism believed current arrangements were adequately dealing with these problems. Furthermore, several interviewees suggested that the gaps in training programmes were being exacerbated by a lack of clear career development paths for those entering the specialist workforce.

In the light of the above comments, it was unsurprising that many interviewees also expressed a desire for changes relating to the training of the public health workforce.

Overall, although now more multidisciplinary in nature, the public health community is also more fractured and disunited and faces a persistent lack of clarity about workforce roles. All this supports Hunter and Sengupta's (2004: 4) claim that: "There remain serious concerns over the purpose of public health, and over the capacity of the workforce and its capability to deliver what is required". As Beaglehole and colleagues suggest, and returning to a central theme of the last section, the problems facing the development of an effective, multidisciplinary public health workforce are closely tied to the question of what public health is: "If public health practitioners are to address national and global health challenges effectively ... a clear vision of what public health is, and what it can offer, is required" (Beaglehole et al, 2004: 2084). A failure to achieve this sense of unity will result, Wills and Woodhead (2004) claim, in public health continuing to be marginalised and failing to form the central concern of any of the various professions deemed part of public health.

These issues are by no means unique to this period in time within England (Beaglehole et al, 2004; Scally and Womack 2004; Tilson and Gebbie, 2004). For example, former WHO Director General, Lee Jong-wook, raised similar concerns in the international context:

> ... progress will at best falter if the capacity issues in public health continue to be ignored or downplayed, if the medical dominance of the speciality reasserts itself, or if the absence of a shared set of values hampers an integrated approach across disciplines and agencies. (Jong-wook, 2003)

Similarly, in a recent review of the public health enterprise in the US, Tilson and Berkowitz (2006) cite a range of challenges to public health that overlaps with many of the issues that have been highlighted in England, including a lack of clarity about the public health function and lines of accountability, gaps in competencies, skills and training, and a paucity of good research.

It might be that adopting the concept of a public health system could offer a way of tackling some of these tensions and deficits. It is certainly the case that some kind of new approach is required, since simply revisiting the issues over time and coming up with the same analyses and prescriptions has not yet resulted in significant progress in improving the public's health, despite the mounting challenges facing it. Chapter Two elaborated on what is meant by such a system and outlined how it might be applied, taking advantage of the diverse sectors and range of expertise that are not axiomatically regarded (or that do not regard themselves) as making a major contribution to improving the public's health. Perhaps trying to get agreement on a definition of public health and discussing the public health workforce as if it comprised only those with public health in their job title should give way to a focus on a complex public health system with multiple facets and resources, and to accessing its relevant components according to the particular public health task requiring attention. Indeed, given the difficulties of defining the public health workforce and determining who should be doing what, we should perhaps focus instead on clarifying the nature of the public health system.

Some final reflections on the evolution of the public health function

Looking back on the history of public health covered so far, it is clear that it has been marked by lack of clarity over purpose, location and the composition of the workforce. Adherence to the three domains of public health developed by the Faculty has tended to reinforce and compound these tensions by simply bundling all of them into the remit and job description of various public health practitioners.

Currently, a lack of clarity over the public health function persists with, for example, Crowley and Hunter (2005: 265) claiming that public health is "being interpreted through the narrow prism of ill health and disease". Elsewhere, Hunter (2003: 101) argues that the term 'public health' is itself a handicap, "since it is not recognised outside the NHS and is imbued with medical overtones".

On a practical level, Holland and Stewart (1998) outline three potential options for the location and organisation of the public health function:

- local government
- independent national body
- health service (NHS).

Each model comprises a mix of potential benefits and problems, as Holland and Stewart (1998) explain. On the one hand, for example, the location of public health within local government can lead to a weakening of essential links between those who have access to health information and specialist health knowledge, and those with the main responsibility for the public health function. On the other hand, the location of public health within the health service limits the influence that practitioners are likely to be able to exert over policies relating to wider determinants of health, such as housing and education, although the introduction of joint appointments may assist in overcoming some of the barriers that historically have existed. Furthermore, the location of public health specialists within the NHS has often resulted in their role being concerned rather more with health service planning than with other aspects of public health, as this book describes. Finally, having an independent national body for public health may suppress local innovation. In addition, while theoretically independent, such a body runs a continual risk of being closed down/replaced if its decisions do not fit with the wider political context. The experience of New Zealand's Public Health Commission is salutary in this respect. Established in 1993, it was disbanded only two years later and its functions were reintegrated into the Ministry of Health and regional health authorities due to a combination of "opposing industry (tobacco and alcohol) pressure, bureaucratic rivalry and a ministerial preference for closer proximity of the public health function" (Davis and Lin, 2004: 200). Recent changes mean arrangements in Wales are now similar to the former New Zealand public health commission model, but these changes have not yet been in place long enough usefully to evaluate or reflect on them. Moreover, following a review of the public health system in Wales, it is likely that there will be changes in these arrangements with a termination of the national agency approach to organising the public health function and a strengthening of the function at local level.

Conclusion

Reflecting on this chapter alongside the previous one, our review suggests that a number of persistent and recurring concerns about the public health function and the associated workforce have been evident throughout the period from 1974 to the present day. The following five merit particular attention:

- Lack of agreement over what the public health function comprises involves persistent tensions between its technical-managerial role and its activist role.
- There is no agreed or shared philosophy governing public health activities, with the result that different models of public health compete with each other, resurfacing over time and jostling with each other for positional supremacy, rather than coexisting in a balanced approach.
- A never-ending succession of organisational reforms (especially affecting the NHS) has presented difficulties for staff trying to settle into posts or build supportive relationships. This has posed a particular barrier for the development of cross-agency partnerships.
- There has been an ongoing debate about how the public health workforce is defined and where it should be located. However, there does now appear to be a consensus that shifting the lead for public health from the NHS back to local government would not in itself resolve the complexities that are intrinsic to the public health function, for it is increasingly recognised that the issues facing public health are not resolvable via structural solutions alone, having more to do with disciplinary and political cultures and associated perceptions of responsibility.
- Despite a recent and welcome shift towards a multidisciplinary workforce, the government's efforts to achieve this through altering training programmes have left a gap in terms of agreeing a set of values to unite the public health movement.

FIVE

Current issues in the public health system in England

The last two chapters described the changing public health landscape in England between 1974 and 1997 and post-1997 respectively, noting the key policy and other milestones in this journey as far as these have shaped and impacted on the direction of policy and the composition and configuration of the public health workforce. Such a period of intense activity, especially since 1997, has inevitably resulted in a range of issues and themes that remain alive and largely unresolved. They are explored further in this chapter and are all matters that are influencing an evolving public health system in one form or other, ultimately determining its ability to deliver. The issues on which we focus in this chapter are as follows:

- the nature of policy formation relating to the health of the public;
- markets, competition and choice;
- commissioning for health and wellbeing;
- public health through partnership;
- public involvement.

The remainder of the chapter is structured around these issues and we draw on our interview material to illustrate each as appropriate.

The nature of policy formation relating to the health of the public

A key tension to emerge from our review of the state of the public health system in England is the lack of certainty and agreement about what the thrust of public health policy is, where responsibility for promoting the health of the public across the wider public health system lies and how much importance is attributed to the impact on health of policies in other sectors.

One means of ensuring policy makers from a wide variety of sectors are sufficiently aware of the health consequences of their policies, currently being promoted by the WHO (2008d), is health impact assessment (HIA). It is a key component of the Health in All Policies

(HiAP) strategy adopted by the EU to inform its health strategy (see Chapter Two). The intention of those advocating for HIA to be undertaken across government in the UK is that it provides a means of ensuring potential health impacts are taken into account in all policy decisions, not merely those emanating from the Department of Health. Theoretically, this could help ensure central government provides a more coherent policy steer on public health issues. However, concerns have been raised about whether HIA, which was originally developed to assess local health impacts, can be effectively adapted to national policy-making levels (Hübel and Hedin, 2003; Davenport et al, 2006). Even if HIA does successfully increase cross-departmental awareness of health impacts, it does not necessarily follow that it will affect subsequent decisions, as alternative political priorities may well dominate (an issue that applies also to local health impacts). On this point, it is important to acknowledge that very different forms of impact assessment (IA) are being promoted by business interests that have obvious conflicts with public health aims. For example, from 1995 onwards, large tobacco and chemical companies have been actively promoting business-oriented forms of IA in the UK and EU (Smith et al, 2010, in press). Currently, policy makers in England are required to undertake a generic form of IA for any proposal that imposes or reduces costs on businesses or the third sector, or that imposes costs of more than £5 million on the public sector (Department for Business, Enterprise and Regulatory Reform, undated). HIA is only one of 12 optional specific IAs that officials are encouraged to consider within this system (others relate to business, equality and environmental impacts). It is therefore extremely unclear whether this approach to IA will encourage policy makers to consider health impacts. Reviews of IAs produced through the European Commission's integrated system found health impacts were frequently undervalued and overshadowed by economic concerns (Wilkinson et al, 2004; Salay and Lincoln, 2008; Ståhl, 2009). The Department of Health has recently commissioned a study of English IAs to assess how, if at all, they are affecting policy outcomes with health impacts (Vohra, in process). To date, despite widespread support for HIA within the public health community, there is little evidence to suggest it has been effective in promoting a coherent approach to public health at a central government level.

Within the context of public health policy, questions remain about what the correct balance is between focusing on the wider determinants of health and on individual lifestyle behaviours. The government seems confused and undecided as to where to place most emphasis, a confusion that appears to be reflected among those working in public health at sub-national levels and that weakens the thrust for the formation of healthy public policy. Certainly, the consensus among the individuals working within the current public health system whom we interviewed is that policy emanating from the Department of Health since 1997 had shifted towards a greater focus on individual lifestyles, in keeping with policy developments around choice, personalisation and the construction of service users as customers. Nearly all of the interviewees suggested that the scales currently needed to be rebalanced in favour of interventions focusing on population-level changes, as well as those focusing on individuals. Even where credit was given to the government for its somewhat limited attempts to address the wider determinants of health, disappointment was expressed over the failure openly to promote such policies (for example, attempts to end child poverty through various initiatives such as the minimum wage, tax credits, Sure Start) to the public. Indeed, interviewees seemed to feel that these policies were almost conducted by stealth.

Despite initial commitments to tackling wider determinants in 1997, and recent reports by the Government Office for Science on obesity (Butland et al, 2007) and the WHO Commission on Social Determinants of Health (WHO, 2008a), which both stress the need for action at a social and environmental level, so far the government appears to have been reluctant to act on such advice. The Foresight report on obesity states that:

> ... although personal responsibility plays a crucial part in weight gain, human biology is being overwhelmed by the effects of today's 'obesogenic' environment, with its abundance of energy dense food, motorized transport and sedentary lifestyles. As a result, the people of the UK are inexorably becoming heavier simply by living in the Britain of today. This process has been coined 'passive obesity'. Some members of the population, including the most disadvantaged, are especially vulnerable to the conditions. (Butland et al, 2007: 2)

The WHO Commission on Social Determinants makes a similar point when it states that:

> ... action on the social determinants of health must involve the whole of government, civil society and local communities, business, global fora, and international

agencies. Policies and programmes must embrace all the key sectors of society not just the health sector. (WHO, 2008a: 1)

The Commission asserts that: "the role of governments through public sector action is fundamental to health equity" (WHO, 2008a: 22). Where they fail to act, perhaps because they lack political will, a push from popular action may be in order. "When people organize – come together and build their own organizations and movements – governments and policy-makers respond with social policies" (WHO, 2008a: 35).

The decision to ban smoking in public places, which required leadership from central government, remains something of an exception (unless the makeover of school meals in England in 2007 is included), with far greater efforts tending to be put into encouraging local agencies to act. That said, as noted in the previous chapter, the government responded to the WHO Commission by establishing its own Review on Health Inequalities in England post-2010 to consider what further action might be taken to improve health equity.

The review's final report was published in February 2010 and endorsed the key message from the WHO Commission on the Social Determinants, namely that reducing health inequalities is a matter of fairness and social justice (Marmot Review, 2010). The review argues that health inequalities stemming from income differentials, education, employment and neighbourhood circumstances are not inevitable and can be significantly reduced to the benefit of the whole of society. To achieve its objectives, the review puts forward two policy goals: to create an enabling society that maximises individual and community potential, and to ensure social justice, health and sustainability are at the heart of all policies. For these objectives to be fulfilled, action across the life course is needed, which will entail attending to early child development, work and employment issues, creating and developing healthy and sustainable places and communities, and prioritising prevention and early detection of those conditions strongly related to health inequalities. Securing success in these areas requires attention to delivery systems, as noted in Chapter Four.

The review sets out an ambitious reform agenda and there must be doubt about how far it will succeed with a change of government a possibility and with the country entering an era of austerity in which significant public expenditure reductions can be expected. Putting sustainability and wellbeing before economic growth to bring about a more equal and fair society, as the review advocates, will require a change of course in respect of current economic and political thinking.

Cynics might argue that the review's purpose was to allow ministers to play for time and postpone taking any further action until after the general election expected in May 2010. Given the depth of the economic crisis, it seems that the options for action are strictly limited in any case regardless of who forms the next government.

Following Tony Blair's stint as Prime Minister (from 1997 until 2007), the avalanche of policy initiatives may be slowing under his successor, Gordon Brown. As far as health policy is concerned this may be no bad thing. A capability review of the Department of Health (all central government departments are subject to such reviews) produced a damning verdict on the Department's poor leadership and lack of strategic direction (Cabinet Office, 2007). It concluded that the Department had failed to take key stakeholders with it on its journey of reform, that the reforms themselves seemed to lack a clear road map or destination and that they appeared to have been conceived in separate silos that did not cohere. The review also claimed that, despite government-wide commitments to "evidence-based policy" (Cabinet Office, 1999), the evidence base for many of the changes did not exist and for others it had been ignored or only selectively drawn on.

There are many lessons here from which the Department of Health can learn, but questions about the impacts of the culture of reform and the consequences of the recent style of successive waves of change may merit their own study. Paradoxically, however, this very culture is likely to prevent such a study from being undertaken. Indeed, such a conclusion can be drawn from Greer and Jarman's study of the Department of Health, which examined how it shifted from being a traditional government department focused on health policy to one fixated on management and delivery (Greer and Jarman, 2007). As the authors conclude, the Department of Health's experiences of hiring staff from outside the career civil service structure "will produce a loss of coherence, knowledge, and *esprit de corps* without necessarily improving policy, management, or 'delivery' capacity" (Greer and Jarman, 2007: 29). Moreover, the move towards devolved responsibility and the creation of a less 'hands on' Department may require further changes in its mode of operation, despite widespread acceptance that a period of stability is desirable to produce coherent approaches to health policy.

Much of what the Cabinet Office capability review has to say is of direct relevance to the public health agenda and to the notion of a public health system as we have used the term. The review notes the health risks of modern lifestyles and asserts that the Department "will need to work in closer partnerships with other organisations to meet these challenges and to make its full contribution to broader social policy"

(Cabinet Office, 2007: 15). Of particular relevance to the public health workforce, the review states that meeting the challenge will require "delivery expertise appropriate for this wider environment" (Cabinet Office, 2007: 15). Perhaps most significantly, the review concludes that the Department "has not yet set out a clearly articulated vision for the future of health … and how to get there" (Cabinet Office, 2007: 18). It goes on to claim that: "there is currently no single clear articulation of the way forward for the whole of the NHS, health and well-being agenda. Consequently, staff and stakeholders are unclear about the vision for health and … feel little sense of ownership of it" (Cabinet Office, 2007: 18). Too often, the review claims, the Department operates "as a collection of silos focused on individual activities" (Cabinet Office, 2007: 19) and, as a result, "cross-boundary integration issues are not routinely thought through" (Cabinet Office, 2007: 21). The review is also critical of the absence of front-line staff engagement in the development of policy and suggests that this results in a lack of common ownership over outcomes. In a section focusing on key areas for action, the review insists that the Department needs to construct "a credible picture of how the whole system will make improving health and well-being its primary focus in the future" (Cabinet Office, 2007: 25). All of this supports our suggestion that it might be more useful to begin to think about public health in terms of a system.

The top management team in the Department of Health, comprising the Permanent Secretary, NHS Chief Executive and Chief Medical Officer, acknowledges that the Department needs "to raise its game on staff engagement and corporate leadership" (Cabinet Office, 2007: 7). However, its subsequent response to the capability review contains little of substance and fails to confront many of the specific criticisms (Department of Health, 2007c). Rather, it comprises a lengthy series of actions to be taken over the next year and beyond. Much of its case rests on the Darzi NHS Next Stage Review, which, as was pointed out in Chapter Four, is more concerned with clinical issues than with public health and seeks to place the onus for change and renewal on clinicians working at local levels, shifting the balance of responsibility accordingly. It is clinicians who are expected to lead the drive for improved quality and for a health service aimed at achieving better health outcomes. How exactly the Darzi approach will fare depends on how long ministers are able to exercise a self-denying ordinance, resisting a hands-on approach to policy making. Perhaps coincidentally, perhaps not, Lord Darzi resigned from his junior ministerial post some months after his report, ostensibly to concentrate on his surgical career.

A follow-up Cabinet Office review two years later concluded that while progress had been made to remedy the deficiencies identified, the "improvements made are not yet sufficiently embedded ... [and are] too reliant on certain individuals" (Cabinet Office, 2009: 8). The review also noted that the Department needed "to clarify its strategic narrative for achieving better health and well-being" (Cabinet Office, 2009: 9). It would seem, therefore, that despite some evidence of progress, many of the problems identified in 2007 remain.

The conclusions from both capability reviews and the initial, somewhat general and non-specific response to the first review, have been reported at some length here because they provide an important context against which to assess the material presented in this chapter. They also lend weight to, and are supportive of, many of the emerging themes and issues identified by our interviewees, especially those concerning the government's commitment to public health, to tackling health inequalities and the perception of policy changes in recent years, which are not felt to be coherently aligned but rather seem, in some cases, to be pulling developments in opposing directions.

Policy connectivity and coherence

One of the key problems that interviewees articulated in relation to the current public health system was the lack of connectivity between its different component parts. The lack of joined-up working appears to be evident at a variety of levels of the system, from the absence of policy coherence at central government level, to the difficulty of ensuring all the necessary parties are actively involved in, and committed to, public health activities at local level. As some of our interviewees noted, connecting these issues effectively requires an appropriate incentive structure to be in place.

A significant number of interviewees felt that the recent lack of policy connectivity had resulted in direct tensions. For example:

> SHA: There are a number of different policy initiatives which potentially conflict. For example we've got the drive to reduce inequalities but the drive to improve choice, and they're in direct competition sometimes. Then we've got this strategic commissioning role of PCTs, but then at the same time more locally deterministic commissioning by practice-based commissioners. And then we have a whole range of models of practice-based commissioning emerging, and in some areas GPs are being very innovative, very

> entrepreneurial, and in other areas they're not interested
> at all, and so we're getting a very patchy landscape of how
> things are going. And it's hard to pull all of that together into
> a sort of coherent model for a patch, so it's quite difficult
> to see where it's going to at times.

The disconnect flagged up in this excerpt between, for example, commissioning for health and wellbeing at PCT level and practice-based commissioning on the other is typical of many such remarks. This is, of course, a fast-moving area of policy development and it is quite conceivable that the criticisms of systemic weaknesses in commissioning, particularly in relation to the absence of requisite skills, are being addressed (if they have not already been by the time this book is published). This is certainly the official response from the Department of Health. However, this presents problems for academic researchers and others seeking to evaluate the changes because situations rarely stay still long enough for any assessment to remain valid for long, or even to inform future developments. For example, a critical review of the NHS reforms from the House of Commons Health Committee expressed considerable scepticism about the ability of commissioning to succeed (although it must be acknowledged that it did not examine the issue specifically from the perspective of health improvement or wellbeing). It concluded that, despite the purchasing/commissioning function having been introduced over 20 years ago, "its management continues to be largely passive when active evidence-based contracting is required to improve the quality of patient care" (House of Commons Health Committee, 2009: p 26, para 56). The Committee was also critical of practice-based commissioning, echoing other critics who argue that it has failed to engage doctors and PCTs and that its relationship with world class commissioning by PCTs "remains opaque and needs greater clarification" (House of Commons Health Committee, 2009: p 61, para 4). However, no sooner had this review appeared than the Department of Health and others, such as the *Health Service Journal*, criticised the Committee for resorting to out-of-date evidence and for not examining what was actually happening at the present time (*Health Service Journal*, 2009). These critics claimed that a very different picture would have emerged if these recent developments had been taken into account as significant progress had been made in recent months. Whether or not this is the case, the Committee is not alone in having serious reservations about commissioning and the manner of its implementation. Ham, for instance, observes that "the gap between research evidence and policy does not augur well for the development of commissioning" (Ham, 2007: 3).

A third major policy conflict on which our interviewees focused was that between the incentives to increase choice vis-à-vis the government's existing commitments to reducing health inequalities. These issues are considered further in subsequent sections of this chapter. More specific policy conflicts that a smaller number of interviewees mentioned included: the government's approach to alcohol (especially the relaxation of licensing hours) compared with its public health commitment to reducing excessive alcohol consumption; the 3% productivity requirement being placed on local authorities, which one interviewee thought would conflict with recent attempts to encourage local authorities to play more of a role in public health; the decision to make commitments to particular programmes, such as child-centred health, even though key sections of the relevant workforce, such as health visitors, had been reduced. Concerns were also raised about how best to prioritise across the three domains of the public health function.

The number of potential conflicts between various policy commitments referred to above paints a picture in which it is likely to be difficult for public health professionals to ascertain precisely what their focus should be or predict how the complex array of recent policy initiatives is likely to unfold and impact on their work. The widespread criticisms within our interview data with regards to the lack of policy coherence emanating from the Department of Health support and confirm the Cabinet Office (2007 and 2009) capability reviews described above. These issues were also evident in the findings of an earlier study, noted in the last chapter, exploring what incentives exist for NHS managers to focus on the wider health issues, which was conducted for The King's Fund by Hunter and Marks (2005). It almost goes without saying that, in the ideal public health system, at least as articulated by most of the interviewees we contacted, national policy would be shaped and coordinated in a manner that ensured that public health issues were consistently prioritised across departments. Indeed, such an approach would be in keeping with the HiAP framework adopted by the European Union and described in Chapter Two. Furthermore, public health values and goals would be mainstreamed to the extent that a broad and diffuse workforce would either have some knowledge of the need to focus on public health outcomes or, at the very least, would be encouraged to work in ways that would contribute to, and promote, better public health outcomes.

In addition to providing a context in which public health objectives were more likely to be achievable, several of the interviewees who focused on the need for greater policy coherence suggested that this issue was linked to the ability to create a public health system that was able effectively to grapple with wider social and economic determinants of health. If public health values could be mainstreamed, the hope, to quote one of the interviewees, was that broader (non-health) policies, at the local and national level, could be "public health proofed" and, as the following interviewee outlines, sectors well beyond the usual public health actors could be brought into public health activities:

> DH: I would like to put public health into local authorities and into libraries and into transport policy and ... I would want to say that every local authority should have a public health impact assessment on its transport policy ... I'd like us to be much more rigorous with the manufacturers of foods, so that instead of them just sort of promising to do better about reducing salt and fat and sugar that they actually had to do better.

The mainstreaming of public health goals presupposes that shared public health outcomes and goals can be achieved, even though many of the interviewees did not feel this was currently the case.

Markets, competition and choice

Markets and choice are the twin pillars of the government's public sector reform strategy as it has evolved since 2004. The assumption is that more efficient, effective and responsive delivery of services, both to treat illness and to promote health, can best be achieved through the application of market-style competitive principles. In this respect, health system reform has pursued a similar direction to other sectors, moving away from a model of traditional top-down central planning towards a model that emphasises local responsibility and the importance of diversity. This new model is expected to be stimulated by market-style competitive principles, including the exercise of choice on the part of service users, although the market model of health reform has not been embraced to the same extent by either Scotland or Wales since devolution (Greer, 2005, 2008). The new model is reflected in the separation of the roles of commissioning services and their provision, with the latter having been opened up to a diversity of providers, risking fragmentation of services and a likely reduction in the extent to which they are accountable to the public. The belief (or hope) is that such mechanisms and incentives will result in more effective and efficient provision (Le Grand, 2007a). However, the argument is predicated on the largely untested assumption that all previous reform attempts have either failed (for example, leaving professionals to manage themselves) or have been seriously limited (for example, a top-down, 'terror by target' culture) (Le Grand, 2009). Such views have been challenged (Hunter, 2008, 2009) and most of the individuals we interviewed viewed such changes with a high degree of scepticism, particularly with regard to their likely impact on public health outcomes. While this does not necessarily imply that such changes are defective, if those entrusted with their execution remain to be convinced of their efficacy and worth, it does suggest that the implementation of such policy approaches is likely to be, at the very least, variable.

For choice to be possible and to succeed, we are told, a market embracing a mix of services and providers has to be in place (Department of Health, 2003). The NHS reforms for England are therefore designed to stimulate diversity of provision (both for-profit and not-for-profit) and to bring to bear on public services and their providers some of the approaches and disciplines from the private sector. Quite how such approaches and levers are to work in the context of public health remains problematic and was a source of some confusion and anxiety among many of the people we interviewed. The majority expressed concern that allowing greater choice would most likely widen health inequalities rather than reduce them, as some proponents, including Le Grand (2009), insist. Only a few of our respondents considered choice to be a potential lever to reach the most socially excluded groups and this was often because they conceived of 'choice' in quite different ways from the majority. When it came to choice of service provider, our interviewees were more comfortable with not-for-profit than with for-profit alternatives. However, there remained doubts about whether such a policy was viable or would make that much difference in practice. The notion of the voluntary sector as being a source of innovation and change in the provision of mainstream as opposed to niche services was treated with some scepticism. There was a concern, too, that for real choice to be available there would need to be spare capacity in the system, which seemed to fly in the face of other pressures to become increasingly efficient (although some key advocates of choice, such as Le Grand, regard choice and efficiency as going hand in hand).

As we go on to show, 'choice' is an ambiguous and somewhat slippery term, which is open to differing interpretations. Consequently, interviewees' views on how recent government initiatives to promote choice might impact on public health tended to depend on what they understood the 'choice agenda' to involve. As the following definition attests, there were at least three quite different ways in which interviewees discussed this agenda: first, there was the frequently referred to commitment to increasing choice within the secondary care sector; second, several interviewees described a scenario in which similar choices could be made available for people who wanted to access preventative services, such as smoking cessation; and, third, a smaller number of interviewees suggested there was a need to think about people's choices on a grander scale, for example, in relation to their abilities to make decisions about where to live or work, or what kinds of food they eat. Most of the interviewees focused on the first two understandings, but the following quotation is one of several examples in which interviewees drew on all three ways of thinking about what 'increased choice' might involve:

> SHA: When you say 'choice', you've got to think big here about what the big issues are in the way people live their lives and how this influences choice, and where … the real enablers of that are.

In addition to illustrating the various ways in which interviewees discussed the 'choice agenda' and, therefore, the lack of a clear conception about what such an agenda involves, the above quotation begins to draw out some of the key concerns that interviewees expressed in relation to policy imperatives to 'increase choice'. Many of these focused on perceptions that taking up opportunities to make better choices might be dominated by wealthier (and generally healthier) groups, concerns discussed in more detail immediately below. However, there was also a range of other, less specific, concerns about recent policy emphases on choice and these are explored in the subsequent sub-section. Following this, we go on to explore aspects of the data that provide more positive interpretations of how the choice agenda could be employed to contribute to public health objectives.

Specific concerns about the impact of the choice agenda on health inequalities

Interviewees in every sector we spoke to expressed concern about the impact that increased choice could have on patterns of already widening health inequalities, a concern that has been much discussed in the literature on the topic (House of Commons Public Administration Select Committee, 2005; *Which?*, 2005; Fotaki, 2006; Fotaki et al, 2006;

Le Grand and Hunter, 2006; Le Grand, 2007a, 2007b; Williams et al, 2007; Hunter, 2008, 2009). The crux of these concerns was a belief that those who were already more health aware and those who had the most resources would be more able to benefit from increased choices, or access the better options, than the already socially excluded groups who populate the lower ends of social gradients of health (Dorling et al, 2007). These concerns were expressed by interviewees working in a range of different contexts and levels. For example:

> PCT: My reservation is that choices are more easily made by articulate and well-informed people and that whole business of the inverse care law, where people are able to make demands on the system and make choices all the time, the people least able to make choices end up with the poorest services rather than the other way around.

> Local government: [Increasing choice] is the same thing as focusing on lifestyle actually because it assumes that people are all as able to choose as each other ... and we just know that that's not true. It will be the vocal, Internet-savvy middle classes that will work out the value for them from those agendas and they'll be badgering their GP or whatever about the choice agenda. It's not going to be people who are socially excluded and marginalised and perhaps who don't speak English and so on.

> DH: We've been quite concerned about the choice agenda and we've been working with colleagues that are doing the choice stuff because we think, potentially, choice can widen the health inequalities, because you need to have ... a degree of economic wellbeing to actually take advantage of the choices.

The quotations above, all of which suggest that the government's emphasis on increased choice may be likely to widen health inequalities, demonstrate a remarkable consistency of opinion across sectors and it is notable, as the last extract illustrates, that these concerns extended to individuals working within central government at the Department of Health.

On the other hand, as previously mentioned, a few interviewees believed that the choice agenda had the potential to help reduce health inequalities, especially if the ensuing changes encourage the provision of services that are more able to reach socially excluded communities. For example, several of the interviewees were hopeful that 'third sector' organisations, such as local voluntary groups, would become more involved in the promotion of health among hard-to-reach communities. With the economic recession leading to significant job losses, the expansion of social enterprises may represent a viable alternative form of employment. Social enterprises are already popular with the government as a way of strengthening social capital and improving the health and wellbeing of communities. The potential benefits they offer are therefore considerable. It is also government policy that the third sector should actively help promote greater diversity and competition in the provision of services and this is linked to the stated belief that this will encourage innovation and new solutions to familiar problems (Department of Health, 2005b). Such views, and the adoption of the choice agenda among at least a few of our interviewees, are also in keeping with the views of recent health policy advisers who have exerted considerable influence on the NHS reforms and on the government's thinking, notably Simon Stevens (2004), Paul Corrigan (2007) and Julian Le Grand (2007a, 2007b). However, the shift from directly provided mainstream services to encouraging social enterprises may, in reality, lead to a greater preponderance of private sector providers, given ambiguities of definition and a blurring of boundaries between social enterprises, large charities, responsible businesses and any kind of mutual association with an interest in health and social care (Marks and Hunter, 2007).

Government policy has become confused on the issue of increasing provider diversity following a speech delivered by the current Health Secretary (at the time of going to press) in which he announced a shift in policy whereby the NHS would become the preferred provider, only putting services out to tender as a last resort (Burnham, 2009). Critics say this marks a reversal of the government's modernisation reform agenda (Corrigan, 2009).

General concerns with the choice agenda

In addition to the potential for increased choice to exacerbate the existing social gradients in health, several interviewees were particularly concerned about what they viewed as increasing encouragement of the for-profit, independent sector to play more of a role in the public health field. As the following quotation reflects, there was a significant level of suspicion among some interviewees about the intentions and motivations of independent sector organisations that have signed up to public health commitments:

> NGO: There is this naivety, as if some of the independent sector's in this ... for philanthropic reasons, to make the health of the public better. Well, I, frankly, struggle to believe that. ... I mean what the independent sector won't be interested in doing is promoting healthier lifestyles unless there's some payoff for it in terms of profit ... And so the notion that Tesco's, for example ... suddenly want to ... put labelling on the ready meals about salt intake and calorific values and so on, they're only doing that because they actually recognise that there's money to be made from doing it. I don't believe that they're in it to make people healthier.

While some interviewees clearly felt that the independent sector had a lot to offer those working towards the achievement of public heath goals, in general interviewees were rather more comfortable with the potential for the third sector to play an increased role in public health, especially in regard to helping more socially excluded groups access health-related programmes. However, in keeping with a recent study of the development of social enterprises in health and social care (Marks and Hunter, 2007), other interviewees felt that the capacity in the third sector for providing a significant amount of health services was minimal. Additionally, some interviewees felt that the government's commitment to increase choice had so far resulted in rather more effort to engage with the independent sector than with voluntary groups and that a level playing field could hardly be said to exist.

One interviewee said s/he felt there was no evidence to suggest that the voluntary sector was likely to provide services any differently from existing providers and therefore that it was unlikely to contribute much to addressing public health issues. A couple of other interviewees, including the following individual, expressed concerns that the third sector would be used as a cheap means of providing existing health services rather than as a source of innovation and a force for change:

> NGO [different interviewee from above]: My fear is that the third sector will be seen as being a cheaper source of resource and actually we will engage with them and commission from them not because what they can do is better or more appropriate or more effective but because it's just cheaper than buying it from the NHS.

Overall, there seemed to be some level of uncertainty and confusion among public health professionals about what the 'third sector' had to offer, or even which kinds of organisations it consisted of. While some interviewees focused on the potential role of the voluntary sector and charitable organisations, others mentioned social enterprises and social marketing organisations in this context, reflecting the wide variety of terms now used in discussions about the 'third sector'.

Other concerns about the choice agenda related to a perceived lack of potential providers to meet many of the service needs, especially in areas that are already relatively underserved. For some interviewees, the choice agenda was perceived to be a potential drain on precious resources that might otherwise be used to achieve public health objectives. For example:

> PCT: I think [the likely impact of the choice agenda is] at best neutral, but quite possibly damaging to public health because … you can only provide choice in a system by having an excess of capacity, so it'll make the provision of health services more expensive. And there's also a need for having additional management capacity to manage choice. So, potentially, what this is doing is using some of the additional resources made available to the NHS to support the whole choice agenda, which could otherwise be used for public health.

The above interviewee's concerns contrast directly with Le Grand's (2007a, 2007b) claims that introducing choice and competition into public services works to increase efficiency and improve delivery. This difference of opinion underlines the varying ways in which individuals expect the choice agenda to unfold.

Positive comments about the choice agenda

Beyond the concerns discussed above, there was a significant level of support for increasing the choices of both commissioners and service users. As with many of the other policy developments that are currently unfolding, there were few unqualified statements of support for increasing choice; most interviewees' enthusiasm was very much dependent on how they believed things might develop. However, for a few of the interviewees, such as the following individual, there was a sense in which the basic concept that 'everyone should have a choice' was something they found inherently attractive:

SHA: Choice has become a sort of pejorative term, it's become something that is linked to the independent sector and linked to assumptions about it as a lever for change. For me, shouldn't everybody have a choice to make about what happens to them and their bodies and their health? ... Some of the most powerful conversations I've had have been around people in the most disadvantaged circumstances saying, "it's my life and I want to be able to choose". But part of ... the problem we have is that we haven't enabled people to have that chance, as a system we haven't necessarily made it possible.

Yet, as the above quotation illustrates, this essentially unqualified support for increasing choice was dependent on a particular interpretation of the choice agenda, one that would require far more than an increase in provider diversity of health services. For enabling people to have real choices may require addressing some of the constraining factors in their social and/or economic circumstances as well as providing a variety of intervention options.

Other comments that were supportive of the general ethos of increasing choice were all also highly dependent on the way in which 'choice' was interpreted, as the following quotation demonstrates:

DH: I think it [the choice agenda] potentially can be quite beneficial. Whether it will be, again, depends upon how it plays itself through because people actually sometimes pay lip service to the words and don't necessarily understand the underlying principles. I would struggle with people who got terribly excited about this and say it's wicked because poor people don't have choice. That's precisely why you have a choice agenda because, actually, what we need to do is to create more opportunity for people to exercise choice than has existed previously, and that's been, for me, the sort of primary reason for adopting policies that are encouraging creative opportunities for choice. But, again, I think it's matching the ambition and the rhetoric with the skills and the understanding to deliver it.

The extent to which interviewees' interpretations of the choice agenda varied is understandable in the light of two issues already raised in this review: the lack of clear policy guidance provided for those individuals and organisations expected to implement central government directives;

and the confused and disjointed broader policy context. The lack of clarity about what the choice agenda entails suggests a more conceptually coherent policy is required before it becomes meaningful for people.

Commissioning for health and wellbeing

Commissioning for health and wellbeing is a third significant development that is of ongoing importance. Since our interviews, there have been a number of initiatives in this area, including the development of organisational competencies for commissioning (Department of Health, 2007e), an assurance framework for PCTs in England based on these competencies (Department of Health, 2008b) and the development of a joint strategic needs assessment (JSNA) for each local authority area, intended to inform commissioning intentions. With its audacious branding as 'world class commissioning', the new approach is widely regarded as critical if there is to be real change and a focus on health outcomes, although whether it, and the initiatives it has spawned, will succeed when it has so far (that is, since the 1990s when first introduced as part of the Conservative government's internal market reforms) failed remains to be seen. To date, the evidence suggests that commissioning remains weak and undeveloped, and is failing to fulfil its potential (Audit Commission and Healthcare Commission, 2008; House of Commons Health Committee, 2009). The Audit Commission's stocktake of progress with the NHS reforms concluded that: "more work is needed to strengthen commissioning" since, without it, "the reform programme will not succeed" (Audit Commission and Healthcare Commission, 2008: 29). For its part, the Health Committee was told by one respected witness that PCT commissioning was the "weakest link of the NHS". The Committee, as was noted earlier in the chapter, remained unimpressed by efforts to strengthen commissioning,.

Commissioning, as in the case of the choice agenda described above, currently remains a largely untested activity with variation among PCTs in how well it is being put into practice and in the extent of public health influence. Certainly, many of our interviewees struggled with the concept, believing it had more to do with purchasing secondary care than with promoting health and wellbeing. While the priority attached to commissioning has accelerated since the publication of the Commissioning Framework for Health and Wellbeing in March 2007 (Department of Health, 2007d) and since we conducted the interviews later that year, it nevertheless remains a concern in some quarters. The arrival of the JSNA may serve to rebalance the agenda in time but, despite promising signs of progress in respect of improving health outcomes, it is too soon to know (Hughes, 2009). In principle, joint commissioning for health and wellbeing (between the NHS and local government) was supported by some of our respondents, although this remains largely uncharted territory and therefore gives rise to particular uncertainty. Nevertheless, closer joint working between the NHS and local government seems likely in future and has been given further endorsement by the emergence of DsPH posts that are jointly appointed between PCTs and local authorities, although what is meant by 'joint' is open to considerable interpretation (Hunter, ed, 2008).

Several of the interviewees had difficulties with the basic concept of 'commissioning for health and wellbeing'. This may seem odd, given that commissioning is ostensibly about improving health outcomes but, for these interviewees, commissioning was an activity that they associated with the provision of health care services and therefore was not one that they felt particularly comfortable using in relation to what they saw as an activity primarily relating to preventative action. In the context of PCTs, this conclusion seems out of kilter with their core business, which is to assess and meet the health needs of their populations, although, as illustrated later, it may simply reflect the fact that factors influencing the broader determinants of health and wellbeing cannot be 'purchased' in a straightforward manner. As the following quotations show, there was a level of resistance to applying the term 'commissioning' to any aspects of public health:

> NGO: How do you commission for [public health], other than commissioning a whole load of health trainers or health promoters or doctors that get a bit more in their contract for doing a bit more blood pressure? … Commissioning … is a totally NHS-based activity … The mere language is exclusive.

> NGO [different interviewee from above]: [Y]ou might want to ask the question whether it's a fundamental dichotomy between the word 'commissioning' and the word 'health improvement', you know? Do we not improve health by other means?

One aspect of joint commissioning that did seem to be welcomed by most interviewees was the role that it was seen to play in promoting collaborative working, particularly between PCTs and local authorities. Additionally, as the next quotation illustrates, some of the interviewees felt that joint commissioning was contributing to improving local flexibility in public health decision making, an aspiration that was also widely supported among interviewees:

> NGO: I think the notion that somehow you can rearrange the pieces locally and you can invest and disinvest according to what is needed, and you have some local latitude over what the priorities are and how things can be done and structured, then I think that, in essence, is a good thing.

Overall, however, there was only a handful of unqualified statements of support for joint commissioning for health and wellbeing within the interview data. This is perhaps not surprising, given that the agenda is so new and had not fully developed or had a chance to bed down at the time of the interviews. It was nevertheless rather worrying, especially in the light of the commissioning framework described earlier, that the data also revealed a lack of clarity about what commissioning involved, with a number of interviewees expressing concerns about the limited guidance on joint commissioning that had been provided to local bodies. These concerns were articulated most clearly by the following interviewee, a director of public health, but were evident in less overt ways in the transcripts of practitioners situated in a range of professional locations:

> PCT: I have a feeling that there's this perplexity around joint commissioning. What does it mean? How are we going to do it? Never mind how are we going to do it in a way that addresses the choice agenda at the same time?

Several factors were perceived by significant numbers of interviewees to be central to the success of commissioning for public health and four in particular merit further attention: first, the development of a workforce equipped with the requisite skills; second, the provision of sufficient resources; third, the achievement of more effective collaborative working; and, fourth, the provision of a coherent and supportive policy context. Each of these factors is briefly discussed in turn, although it should also be acknowledged that several additional factors were perceived to be important by a smaller number of interviewees, including: the use of available evidence in making decisions about commissioning; organisational and policy stability; and increased public awareness of public health aims and involvement in commissioning.

The development of a workforce equipped with the requisite skills

Bearing in mind that commissioning for health and wellbeing is a relatively recent policy initiative, it is not surprising that many of the skills required for it have not formed part of public health specialists' training to date. Several interviewees felt this consequent lack of skills posed a threat to the potential success of the commissioning agenda:

> PCT: Commissioning did not go well at all [in this area]... and the reason for that was, certainly here, we're up against the might of hospital trusts and, being smaller PCTs with ... less skilled people, we weren't effective at all.

> NGO: One of the problems is there's a lack of commissioning experience in the public health community. We found this when recruiting directors of public health. We couldn't find enough individuals who are really good at this, even for the NHS side of things. To find those who have got any experience of commissioning, more broadly, in social care environments, for example, is very rare. And so we've got a workforce which may not have all the skills it needs to deliver on this agenda.

Several of the interviewees based in the Department of Health accepted that a lack of capacity and skills was a problem that the commissioning agenda, and public health more generally, faced. However, they were, overall, more optimistic than many of the other interviewees that current and planned investments in training and capacity would overcome these difficulties. Some of the interviewees based in public health specialist posts framed the problem of a lack of skills relating to commissioning as part of a more general predicament caused by constant policy change (an issue already touched on earlier and discussed further below). In addition, there is a danger that the public health potential of the commissioning agenda, which after all has the byline "adding life to years and years to life", is thwarted to the extent that DsPH take a back seat and/or fail to implement a public health model of commissioning. Long-standing, and well-documented, weaknesses in public health leadership tend to confirm that it is a well-founded concern (Alderslade and Hunter, 1994; Nutbeam and Wise, 2002; Hunter, ed, 2007a; Hannaway, 2008).

The provision of sufficient resources

As with many new initiatives, there were concerns expressed among those expected to implement policy directives around joint commissioning that a lack of resources may also hamper success. For many of the interviewees, this wariness arose within a context in which public health frequently loses funding to other parts of the health system (as discussed in Chapter One). Many of the interviewees were therefore quite pessimistic about the likelihood that this issue would be effectively resolved, as the following quotation illustrates:

> DH: You've always got the barrier that there's never enough money to do any of this sort of stuff ... particularly as we're into much tighter financial regimes from now on, and there'll be the usual scrabbling around in public health ... actually trying to get the resources.

However, some of the interviewees, particularly RDsPH and those based at the Department of Health, were keen to emphasise that a focus on limited funding should not be seen as an excuse for a lack of achievement of public health outcomes. Several examples of low-cost initiatives that were perceived to be effective were cited as evidence that limited resources did not necessarily pose a barrier.

The achievement of more collaborative working

Although, as already discussed, policy imperatives for joint commissioning for health and wellbeing were perceived to aid the development of public health partnerships, the barriers to effective collaboration were also viewed by many of the interviewees as a potential threat to the success of commissioning. In the following quotation, a range of problems facing partnership working is highlighted, including confusion around which organisations are responsible for which aspects of commissioning, and conflicts between different organisational approaches, both of which the interviewees suggested were exacerbated by a lack of clear guidance from central government:

> NGO: Local authorities have got a great history of public health improvement, and they see themselves often as the lead public health agency, and quite rightly in many cases, but, unfortunately, so do the NHS. And so the

new commissioning framework, I don't think it's a good document, I think it's a bit woolly, and it doesn't make the accountabilities and the priorities very clear. And what's happening already is that directors of adult social services and children's services are running off with this agenda in one direction with local authority executives, and public health directors are running off in another.

Some interviewees felt, for joint commissioning to be truly effective, there was a need not only for far clearer guidance for those involved but also for organisational arrangements and performance assessment mechanisms to be brought into line with each other (an issue touched on earlier in this book). In fact, as the following sub-section discusses, many of the interviewees suggested that, rather than providing clear guidance, some other recent policy initiatives emanating from central government appeared directly to conflict with the aims of commissioning for health and wellbeing.

The provision of a coherent and supportive policy context

Much of the cautiousness surrounding commissioning for health and wellbeing seemed to relate to many interviewees' concern that, while potentially useful, it was not an approach that they felt would, in itself, solve many of the problems that were currently facing public health. Or, as one RDPH summed it up, "it's only one bit of the jigsaw". Hence, many interviewees felt that, in order to be successful, the commissioning framework needed to be underpinned and accompanied by clearer directives and incentives for local actors to work with:

> DH: I think it will be successful but not necessarily as successful as it could be. I think there are still issues about the need to raise awareness and create better understanding of the reasons why people should be interested in this ... When you work in partnership in the messy world of management, what you learn very quickly is that you actually have to understand the motives of individuals and how you can motivate people to take on board an agenda.

In addition, many of the interviewees were frustrated by the lack of coherence between the commissioning agenda and various other recent policy initiatives. For example:

DH: I think some of the building blocks work against each other. For example ... we've set up something that's called payment by results – it isn't really payment by results, it's payment by activity – and we're not really thinking about the desirable outcomes. What we want is hospital services that will take pride in the fact that patients don't need to come to them again and will support what goes on in the community because that's the right thing to do. So there are bits of the system that are working against each other. Demand management in primary care versus the magnet effect of the big hospital.

As discussed earlier in relation to general concerns about a lack of policy coherence within public health, practice-based commissioning (PbC) was the policy most often highlighted by interviewees as one that seemed potentially to conflict with the aims of joint commissioning for reasons to do with both scale and inclination. Several interviewees felt that PbC functioned at a level and scale that rendered joint commissioning virtually impossible and pointed out that, even if it could be made to work, most GPs have no experience or understanding of working with local government and little if any enthusiasm for such a task.

Relating to the concerns discussed above, several interviewees were keen to suggest that, if commissioning for health and wellbeing were to be successful, it would need to be given space and stability to develop effectively. These comments were often made in the context of frustrations about the raft of recent reorganisations:

NGO: I think it mustn't become a political whim that's swept away should we have a new kind of political administration, because I think it has to have some longevity, it has to really have time to bed in properly.

This finding is indicative of the fact that, despite the expression of a range of reservations about recent developments in public health, including the commissioning agenda, nearly all of the interviewees advocated a period of 'bedding down' in public health, in which they could concentrate on trying to implement recent policies effectively rather than having to understand new initiatives.

The importance of basing public health decisions on available evidence and information was an issue that interviewees raised in a range of contexts but, to several interviewees this seemed to be particularly significant in regard to local decision making around commissioning activities:

> NGO: I think if people really wanted that to happen then it could do, but it has to be absolutely embedded across the system, so that when people are making decisions about commissioning the very first thing they ask is "what do we know about existing services? What data have we got? What evidence have we got about whether they're working or not? What evidence is there around about whether there's a more cost-effective way of doing things?"

As the above quotation indicates, comments about the need to base decisions on evidence were usually made in the context of suggestions that this was far from the current reality. Indeed, some interviewees suggested that it was difficult to obtain the kinds of information they required to make decisions about commissioning. All this suggests that, despite official commitment to the idea that policy and practice should be based on information about 'what works', the current reality is a long way from evidence-based (or even informed) policy and practice.

The final factor that several interviewees suggested was essential if commissioning for health and wellbeing was to succeed was an increased awareness of public health issues among the general population, as the following interviewee articulated:

> SHA: I think it's about the role the public should be playing in terms of influencing commissioning, full stop, and the fact is that people are interested in their health. We ought to engage the public much more in thinking about the broader aspects of public health policy, but that does require us to take the agenda to the public in a way that we don't do at the moment.

Commissioning for health and wellbeing, like many other public health initiatives, was thought to be more easily achievable in a context in which the public were more involved in and more committed to public health goals. While this seems reasonable, there were a number of concerns about how the goal of increased public awareness and involvement might be achieved, a point discussed further below.

Public health through partnership

An abiding theme of policy and practice for many years, but especially over the past decade or so, has been the importance of partnerships to achieve objectives in complex systems that straddle several organisations and policy sectors (Smith et al, 2009). In addition to being an activity that many interviewees felt was being actively promoted by the commissioning agenda for health and wellbeing, effective partnership working is something that the three post-1997 Labour governments have promoted as being of central value to public health in its own right.

With a clearer acknowledgement of the role of the wider determinants of health, especially during the early years of New Labour, the policy context was actively promoting notions of 'cross-sectoral', 'joined-up' and 'partnership' working, as well as placing significant emphasis on public involvement and accountability (for example, Cabinet Office, 1999). From a public health perspective, this resulted in a renewed focus on projects that sought to involve and empower communities, as well as a series of policy initiatives designed to promote partnership working, both within the NHS and between the NHS and other organisations.

Various provisions to encourage joint working, including pooled budgets, were made in the 1999 Health Act. There was also a range of initiatives designed to promote partnership working, such as health action zones and health improvement programmes (see Chapter Four, Box 4.2), plus a specific charge on PCTs to promote partnership working. The 2000 Local Government Act gave local authorities the power to promote social, economic and environmental wellbeing, placing a renewed emphasis on the role that local government should play in promoting public health. Since then, support for jointly appointed directors of public health has emerged and most appointments at this level are now 'joint', although, as noted above, not without some concerns about what it is they are intended to achieve and by what means (Hunter, ed, 2008).

The interviewees' comments suggest that efforts to strengthen partnerships are widely supported among those working to implement policy change, but that they have so far met with mixed success. While some interviewees reported extremely positive accounts of partnership working in their locality (or region), through LSPs and other arrangements, there were also a few very negative accounts. Overall, the most frequent response was to suggest that efforts had clearly been more fruitful in some areas than others, as the following extract attests:

NGO: I think it [partnership working] is inconsistent across the country. I think where there's been a history of people working together, perhaps even before we started formally calling it partnership, but actually where people have been in the same local place and have been kicking around for 20 or 25 years and have been getting things done, then actually I think they do seem to work. And they've got some maturity and there's some respect and some trust and they're focused. I think where they've been flung together because there's an imperative to do so, but actually that people don't really understand what it is that they're supposed to be doing, they don't really feel any confidence in terms of if they have any clout locally to make things happen, then I think partnerships don't work, frankly.

Several of the factors interviewees deemed important in determining the success (or otherwise) of partnership working are mentioned in the above quotations, including the extent to which partner organisations (and individuals) had previously worked together, the level of trust/ antagonism between partners and arrangements relating to resources. Other factors that interviewees suggested impacted significantly on the effectiveness of efforts to promote partnership working included whether or not boundaries between partnership organisations were coterminous and whether partnerships shared the same targets, incentives and performance assessment arrangements. Each of these factors is now briefly explored in turn.

The extent to which partner organisations (and individuals) have historically worked together

As the previous quotation demonstrates, a history of partnership working was often seen as a key factor determining the success of current attempts to work collaboratively. Where organisations had previously worked together, many interviewees suggested this had allowed structures to develop that helped promote ongoing efforts to collaborate and often resulted in a perception that working jointly was the norm, rather than something that had to be worked towards:

Local government: [Partnership working here] really has had a lot of time to form and [is the] norm and all those things. So it's had a lot of time to embed itself, and so its history is very important. And I think sometimes we sort

of gloss over the importance of people who know each
other quite well and have worked together for some time
as giving you a very strong foundation.

Additionally, interviewees suggested that a successful history of
partnership working was often associated with sound levels of shared
knowledge between different partner organisations and a level of trust
that could not necessarily be quickly developed. As the following
sub-section discusses, a relationship of mutual trust between partner
organisations was considered to be extremely important in making
collaborative working effective.

The level of trust/antagonism between partners

The extent to which people working within different organisations
feel that they can work with one another, and the extent to which they
trust both the partner organisation and the individuals who work for
it, were viewed by many of the interviewees as crucial to the efficacy
of organisational relationships, as the following interviewee reflects:

> DH: I think it goes back to the fact that they think it's an
> important set of longer-term objectives for their area, and
> they like working with each other. I don't think it's the
> form of organisation and I don't really, deep down, think it's
> even the money ... I think it's about whether people can
> settle as an effective working network. A focus on outcomes
> I think is perhaps the one thing I would say that is really
> important. A lot of people go through the ticking the box
> ritual ... It needs more than that.

The difficulty with focusing on issues such as the level of trust between
organisations and the importance of having a history of partnership
working is that these are not factors that can readily be replicated.
Furthermore, it would be difficult to design a policy that had the specific
aim of developing trust between several types of organisation, as the
key determinants of trust are likely to be specific to different contexts.
Therefore, while many of the interviewees suggested these issues were
important, they were not necessarily the issues that interviewees felt
policy makers ought to be addressing as a means of helping collaborative
working to take root.

Coterminosity of boundaries across organisations

In contrast, coterminosity of boundaries between partner organisations, a subject that arose in every interview, was precisely such an issue. While several of the interviewees suggested that it was important not to overemphasise the benefits of coterminosity, or conclude that effective partnership working was impossible without it, no one thought it was irrelevant and many, such as the following interviewees, believed it was crucial:

> DH: I think, generally speaking, coterminosity can only be good, if only because the players sitting around the table are actually focused on the same area and on the same problems.

> PCT: I think [coterminosity of boundaries] is, having got that now, we haven't had it for five years, it's really important. It's vital, really. I mean ... it is so much harder to work when you're not coterminous.

Most of the interviewees, including those quoted here, discussed coterminosity in relation to the local level (between PCTs and local authorities) and it was at the local level that coterminosity was deemed by many to be essential to effective partnership working. However, where coterminosity of boundaries at the regional level was discussed, interviewees generally felt this was also important.

Yet, while nearly all of the interviewees were in favour of achieving coterminosity of boundaries (at the local level, at least), the high levels of resistance to further organisational restructuring suggest a desire for sharing boundaries was not of paramount importance and not something interviewees felt ought to be achieved at any cost, especially as the recent raft of organisational reforms was suggested by many interviewees to have been extremely damaging to relationships between PCTs and local authorities.

Shared targets, incentives and performance assessment arrangements

As already discussed, one of the key factors that many interviewees felt policy directives ought to be more effective in encouraging was the development of shared incentives, targets and goals to work towards. A positive example, where several interviewees suggested this had recently occurred, was around smoke-free initiatives. For example:

> PCT: I think one thing that is galvanising us all is the smoke-free agenda. I mean that's great, but then that timetable is driven nationally by everybody, and that has brought a lot of people together. So it's been fantastic because everybody has to do something by the 1st of July, and we are important players because we have the smoking cessation services, and that has been a really very interesting one. So in a way maybe it needs something of that sort to bring it all together and, if you can find something else where you've got that sort of deadline, then it might galvanise action that would otherwise just drag on.

In addition to a perceived need for joint targets and goals, several of the interviewees felt it was necessary to link the currently separate performance management systems governing local authorities and PCTs together. The comprehensive area assessments (CAAs) introduced in 2009 are intended to go some way towards doing precisely this by taking a more holistic view of a local area and by embracing both local government's and PCTs' contributions to improved health and wellbeing. Moreover, mindful of the need to avoid separate audits in public health, where there was much overlap between the work of the Audit Commission and former Healthcare Commission, the two bodies established a close working relationship and undertook several joint reviews over the lifetime of the Healthcare Commission between 2004 and 2009. However, with the demise of the Healthcare Commission in April 2009 and its replacement by the Care Quality Commission, it is not yet clear whether this joined-up approach will be maintained in future.

Arrangements relating to resources

The provision of joint targets and performance assessment mechanisms was not the only area that many of the interviewees felt ought to be shared across organisations. The separate budgets for contributing to public health initiatives held by local authorities and PCTs were thought by several interviewees to hinder collaborative working. In the following extracts, the first interviewee was reflecting on his/her suspicion that he/she could work more effectively as a *joint* DPH if the local authority contributed to funding his/her post. The second quotation refers to funding issues more generally:

> PCT: I can see that logically joint funding might make a difference because, if the local authority were paying half of my salary, I suspect that I'd be held to account rather more rigorously by the local authority than is the case at the moment. I mean, ideally, I would like to say that it doesn't make any difference but, in practice, I think it does.

> SHA: At the moment though, even within the LAA, my understanding is that the funding still comes down relevant government department streams. But, if they move to the next step and actually say, "here is a pot of money and it's for all of the agencies", that's going to create a new dynamic of people really having to get into conversations about who gets the investment and why.

For many interviewees, local area agreements (LAAs) and joint DPH posts both represented moves towards better linking of funding and priorities across local authorities and PCTs, and many were hopeful that these moves would contribute a great deal towards effective partnership working and the achievement of better health outcomes. Joint DPH posts pose a number of issues that are considered by Elson (2008) in a critical review of their roles. Nevertheless, such posts have been generally welcomed, although with a preference for putting them on a firmer statutory basis "making clear the roles, responsibilities and reporting lines" (Local Government Association, 2008: p 107, para 6.42), points reflected in our interviews.

LAAs were particularly perceived by interviewees to represent an extremely positive development within public health. Most were optimistic that they would help promote joint planning and would provide mechanisms for linking incentives and rewards across local authorities and PCTs, as the following quotations demonstrate:

> SHA: I think local area agreements are brilliant and are going extremely well ... The LAAs have very heavy – very substantial in some cases – reward grants associated with them. So putting together a good LAA with a high health content and significant sums of money flowing from that, I think is quite an incentive for good partnership work.

DH: [LAAs are] fundamental. This is the actual mechanism for really bringing organisations together much more powerfully than tinkering around with the organisational form. The local area agreements are rapidly becoming the centre of the contract with central government ... Too many of the partnerships at the moment are not connected to the outcome side, and the LAA I think connects it to the outcomes.

In fact, aside from one RDPH's concerns about the increased bureaucracy that the implementation of LAAs had brought to his/her region, one of several negative comments regarding LAAs related to the possibility that the constantly shifting policy environment, combined with the limited resources available within public health, might mean that they were prevented from achieving their full potential. The Institute for Government (IfG), in a study of "the art of performance management" also found wide support for LAAs with evidence of "green shoots of progress" (Gash et al, 2008: 8). However, it remains the case at the time of writing that much of the progress that has been welcomed relates simply to developing new relationships, although it has also been claimed that "discussions are already beginning to improve understanding of the interconnectedness of a wide range of problems" (Gash et al, 2008: 8). There is also early evidence of LAAs allegedly resulting in small-scale local innovations, although whether these can become scaled up to meet the challenges in areas like childhood obesity and teenage pregnancy is less certain. At the same time, there is anecdotal evidence that is less encouraging and shows central government departments seeking to influence LAAs and determine their priorities.

While LAAs may be generally supported and have already given rise to some significant positives, they are not a complete success story. The IfG's comments on LAAs included that the LAA process remained bureaucratic and burdensome, with new indicators being added on top of existing ones. It was also claimed that LAA activity "was not translating into action at the rate that many had hoped" (Gash et al, 2008: 9). There was little evidence of widespread innovation and no examples of significant increases in pooled budgets for cross-agency initiatives. (see also a review of pooled budgets by the Audit Commission, 2009). In addition, the process of selecting LAA priorities did not always tie in with other local area strategies. Moreover, the timing of the agreed LAA priorities meant that they would not impact on budgets until April 2009, some ten months after they were signed off. So, at least for the time being, the jury is out in respect of how effective LAAs will prove to be. The CAAs, referred to earlier in this chapter, may be critical in terms of exerting pressure on all local agencies to ensure that LAA priorities are achieved. Whether CAAs will be able to meet such expectations remains uncertain. Indeed, the tendency of new arrangements like LAAs and CAAs to over-promise is a real danger as it paves the way for potential disillusionment and consequential cynicism. Compounding this problem, weak cross-departmental working in Whitehall continues and inevitably imposes limits on how far joined-up activity can be achieved and sustained locally. Once again, the prospect of further organisational reforms, especially in the light of the economic recession and need for stringent public spending cuts, poses potential problems; if LAAs are to succeed, they need to be given time to prove themselves but recent history suggests this kind of space is rarely provided, and a further round of reform is likely. History tells us that 'quangos' (quasi non-governmental organisations) are easy prey for governments in search of efficiency savings. As far as the NHS is concerned, a cull of SHAs and PCTs is a clear possibility. Like many of our interviewees, the Local Government Association (LGA) wants to see LAAs and LSPs strengthened in order to improve local accountability for public health (Local Government Association, 2008), which might take the form of creating a clearer statutory duty on the LAAs' partners to work together to improve the public's health. However, at the end of the day, LAAs, LSPs and other arrangements merit continuing support only if they result in better public health outcomes, something that it has yet to be proven that partnership working can deliver (Smith et al, 2009; Perkins et al, 2010).

Public health outcomes

For some interviewees, as several of the quotations in the previous sub-sections suggest, the importance of being able to work collaboratively within the field of public health to improve health outcomes seemed intuitive due to the complex and multifarious nature of the factors that influence health. However, other interviewees were keen to emphasise that being able to work effectively in organisational partnerships did not automatically mean that different, or better, health outcomes would be achieved:

> SHA: Most local area agreements are lists of what the partners were going to do anyway on their own. So they are not, there isn't added value to be seen from the partnership ... If partnership working is part of the evidence base and part of the rigour with which you would pursue your target then that's appropriate, but it isn't an outcome in its own right. Sometimes the topic itself doesn't have the necessary evidence that a partnership will make the blind bit of difference, so why would you have one?

> PCT: It's very unpolitically correct for me to say so really [but] there are some aspects where partnership working is oversold, and you might actually do better on your own without ... coming together.

A couple of other interviewees were also keen to highlight that the desirability of a partnership might depend on the partners involved; not all organisations or sectors were seen in a positive light by all of the interviewees. For example, the following interviewee was rather wary of partnerships that involved the private sector:

> NGO: I think there's a lot of naivety about what partnerships are. For example, particularly with the industry, I think ... there are some inappropriate partnerships in public health which I think are unprofessional and actually damage public health, particularly with commercial interests. I agree with the dialogue with the commercial interests but I think some of the partnerships are not merited ... because the commercial partners haven't [yet] embraced the sort of change [required].

The concerns raised by the above interviewee are reflected in recent unease about the Department of Health's decision to allow several large food corporations, including PepsiCo and Kelloggs, to partially sponsor its three-year 'Change4Life' initiative. The stated aim of government is to ensure the UK becomes "the first major nation to reverse the rising tide of obesity" (Cross-Government Obesity Unit et al, 2008) but a recent editorial in *The Lancet* (Editorial, 2009) argues that the decision to allow companies that "fuel obesity" to become partners in the 'Change4Life' campaign is "ill-judged" and "should have been avoided". It is a view shared by NGOs like the National Heart Forum.

Given that the campaign only commenced in January 2009, it is not yet possible to judge how, if at all, commercial involvement affects its success in this particular example, but it is clear that there are growing concerns about commercial involvement in health policy and governance (see, for example, Buse and Lee, 2005). Within our interview data, tensions about which individuals and organisations different interviewees believed had something positive to contribute to public health were most overt in relation to discussions about recent policy emphases on the importance of choice, as discussed earlier.

Local government and public health

Since 1974, as we discussed in Chapter Three, local government's engagement with the public health agenda has been problematic, often for reasons to do with language and cultural differences, which have, on occasion, led to a virtual stand-off between local authorities and health service organisations (Elson, 1999). Developments in neighbourhood renewal and regeneration, and concern about social exclusion in the late 1990s, have resulted in renewed interest in health issues in local government (Blackman, 2006). Overview and scrutiny committees have sought to look at health issues more broadly, beyond concerns about local hospital closures, and health and wellbeing partnerships are developing joint strategies to improve health and address inequalities. The introduction of terms such as 'wellbeing' and 'social responsibility' are helping to overcome some of the language-related barriers that may have prevented local government from assuming a leadership role in relation to health issues. Nevertheless, for the most part, local government has yet to seize the initiative in respect of public health, even though it is well placed to do so (Elson, 2007).

Notwithstanding a few dissenting voices, the weight of evidence submitted to the Health Committee's 2001 inquiry into public health did not favour returning to a pre-1974 style of organisation for public health (House of Commons Health Committee, 2001a). Rather, in a world of constant change, the challenge was believed to be largely about working together, wherever people are located, and not about changing structures. However, there was support for making a clearer distinction between the public health function and individuals who play a professional role in public health, in part to avoid confusion between responsibility for health services and responsibility for health.

Realising the potential for local government to improve health has become a common refrain but, with health continuing to be seen as the business of the NHS, it has been difficult to sustain a strong leadership role for local government. In theory this is surprising since the list of local government functions and services that act to improve the health and wellbeing of the local population exceeds that of any other public body. However, local government's vital role has been "both obscured and undermined by the policy fragmentation which has separated policy on healthcare from the wide range of policies determining the conditions in which health can be sustained" (Local Government Association et al, 2004: 14).

Importantly, these latter policies "have not enjoyed the same political salience as policies affecting healthcare" (Local Government Association et al, 2004: 14). Such a situation led the Health Committee to conclude that: "local authorities have yet to realise their full potential when it comes to public health" (House of Commons Health Committee, 2001a: para 129). A briefing paper for the Society of Local Authority Chief Executives (SOLACE), released in the same year as the Health Committee report, urged local authorities "to reclaim their original role as champions of the health of local communities" (Duggan, 2001: 2). Yet such a role will not fall to them by default; local authorities "must make the most of their unique position as community leaders to create a vision for health at local level and use their skills and resources to ensure that there is maximum impact on the health of local people" (Duggan, 2001: 2).

The creation of DPH posts that are jointly appointed by PCTs and local authorities has occurred at an increasing pace over the past year or so in England. On the whole, the view held is that such joint appointments are helping to join up the different infrastructures of PCTs and local government, that they provide a bridge across cultural divides and that they are enabling both organisations to understand better those aspects of public health on which they ought to be focusing. However, interviewees also suggested that there were currently a number of factors working to limit the effectiveness of these posts.

The difficulties that interviewees described in relation to the functioning of joint DPH posts related to cultural differences between the NHS and local government, and to unrealistic expectations of such posts if seen in isolation from a joint public health system more generally. Such concerns echoed a variety of the problems facing public health more generally that this book has already touched on, including the barriers to effective partnership working, especially between local authorities and PCTs; the need for a coherent approach to public health, in which the current variety of policies are more closely aligned and interlinked; and a desire for clearer guidance for policy initiatives. This suggests that the difficulties facing those individuals trying to operate effectively as joint DsPH in fact reflect broader problems facing public health, which might best be dealt with by a more widespread review of public health policy and what it is intended to achieve. Certainly, as several of the interviewees made clear, it would be unreasonable to expect the creation of joint DPH posts alone to overcome many of these quite profound problems and tensions, a point made also by Elson (2008) in his critique of joint DsPH posts.

Public involvement

As in the case of partnership working, the involvement of the general public in decision making is a development that has been actively encouraged in a range of recent policy statements (for example, Secretary of State for Health, 2004, 2006) and it was similarly a trend often discussed by interviewees as being an intrinsically valuable objective. However, there is evidence that, in practice, effective public involvement continues to elude public health. For example, a research project entitled 'Strategic action programme for healthy communities' (Pickin et al, 2002) identified a lack of a strategic approach to working with communities and explored the organisational changes required in the public sector if the commitment to developing more effective partnerships with the community was to be achieved. Public sector organisations found it hard to engage with communities for a number of reasons, including: the community's capacity to engage; the skills and competencies of staff within organisations; the professional service culture; the overall organisational ethos; and the dynamics of local and national political systems. Other research demonstrates that collaboration and partnership with the voluntary and community sectors is effective for building community relationships (Farrell, 2004). With the creation of local involvement networks (LINks) in every local authority area in 2008 (following the 2007 Local Government and Public Involvement in Health Act) it is hoped that local communities will be able to exert more influence on local public services. However, it remains to be seen whether the removal of responsibility for patient involvement from the patient and public involvement forums of the NHS to LINks (which span health and social care across a local authority area) will be reflected in a broader approach to public health and wellbeing, and whether their work will be influenced by the priorities of joint strategic needs assessments.

At the time of the interviews, most of the people we spoke to felt that the public health community had been particularly poor at involving the public in decision making to date. For example:

DH: Many of the people who talk about patient and public involvement, about expert patients, about a patient-led NHS, actually don't get it, because, as soon as patients do start making real choices, we try to stop them again. So we say we want them to do that but we will not follow where they lead. And so my concern is that there's still a kind of paternalistic intent so that, if you like, public engagement becomes a trick instead of a proper intention. It becomes a sort of thought that, "oh well, we can use public engagement just to trick people into doing what we want and what we've decided they ought to do in the first place".

NGO: I think any public health system needs public [and] community involvement, and again I think that's been a real area of weakness in public health systems certainly in recent times ... [The public should have a] much bigger role than the role they've got at the moment would be my view. I think, and local government and the NHS are equally guilty of this, but probably the NHS is a bit more guilty than the local government, they're all 'doing to' organisations.

In addition to suggesting that recent attempts to engage local communities in public health decision making had been rather limited, the above quotations both suggest that there is a tendency within public health for professionals to want to shape public behaviour, rather than be informed by it. There was only limited evidence to support this claim within the interview data but a couple of the DsPH and RDsPH who were interviewed were notably less enthusiastic about public involvement than other interviewees. The following extract is the most overt example of this, in which the interviewee openly reflects on his/her concerns about community involvement:

PCT: I think I know what the priorities should be from the data and so on and, if I involve the public, it's just because I know implementation will be harmed if they don't believe it's their idea in the first place. And that is being deeply cynical isn't it? Because that is not actually saying I want them to come up, naturally, with what the priorities are, I'm saying – because I'm an arrogant sort – that I think I know what the priorities are but I'm going to try to engage them to sort of come up with my priorities. So it is quite difficult because, when you do get public meetings and so on, they keep on focusing down on closure of the acute hospital or ... I mean occasionally there's something that comes up about TB, "all those nasty foreigners bringing that awful disease", and so ... it's embarrassing so you have to put it back into the box.

Another interviewee felt that the public were growing increasingly tired of being asked for their opinions about policy decisions and that the job of local practitioners and central government policy makers should be to make informed decisions in the interests of the population, rather than continually consulting the public about their preferences. While only a small number of interviewees suggested that these were reasons to avoid placing too much emphasis on public involvement, many other interviewees felt they were issues that needed to be confronted if public involvement was going to be successful. Yet, while most interviewees were supportive of the general principle of involving the public more actively in decision making, the data reveal a tangible lack of knowledge about how best to achieve this aim. As the following quotations illustrate, several interviewees were concerned with the ineffectiveness of current arrangements and yet were equally unclear about what better alternatives might involve:

Local government: If you went down a busy street and asked people what they thought about health, they would be likely to talk about hospitals and their Uncle Bob and his experiences – unclean wards or whatever. So you've got a real challenge there. Before you can involve the public effectively in the health and wellbeing agenda, you have to do some education around what that is – about people's health. So that's a fundamental challenge really.

PCT: How do you engage with the public? How do you find out what they think about public health issues and how do you ensure that their comments, their views, are well-informed because, at the end of the day, they're not, Joe Public isn't a public health specialist and so they may come up with things and say things are important that, objectively speaking, aren't. And that's a real challenge.

In addition to the lack of confidence among interviewees in relation to their knowledge of how most effectively to engage the general public in public health agendas, a recurring concern in the interview data in regard to public involvement (and one that is evident in all three of the previous quotations) is that public perceptions of what constitute public health problems are not necessarily the problems on which public health practitioners and policy makers are currently focused. In light of this, several interviewees felt a significant amount of public education was required before the public could be usefully engaged in making decisions about potential public health options. Some of these frustrations are reflected in the limited research that has specifically explored lay perceptions of prominent public health issues. For example, research exploring public perceptions of health inequalities found that, overall, the public do not tend to be overly concerned about health inequalities (Blaxter, 1997) and, furthermore, that the individuals who are most likely to experience the negative effects of health inequality (that is, those living in difficult social or economic circumstances) tend to be more reluctant than others to accept the existence of health inequalities (Popay et al, 2003), possibly due to the stigmatising effect that accepting the existence of health inequalities can have on communities and individuals.

Other concerns that interviewees discussed included uncertainty about how to avoid the trap of having the same, not necessarily representative, groups ('the usual suspects') repeatedly contributing to debates while most of the population remain unengaged, and the difficulties involved in getting the public to think about dealing with potential, rather than actual, health problems. The former is an issue raised by Tritter and Lester (2007) in their recent analysis of how emphases on the importance of user involvement link to the policy priority of tackling health inequalities. Here, they reflect that "patterns of health inequality are also reflected in those who tend to be involved and those who are members of 'hard to reach' groups" and conclude that: "[u]nless user involvement draws on the diverse range of the population and aims to be inclusive, it can only serve to reinforce existing patterns of health inequality" (Tritter and Lester, 2007: 175).

As has already been highlighted, many of the interviewees felt that the public health system ought to engage more effectively with the public. For some, this was one of the ways in which they hoped the public health system would improve over the next five years:

> Local government: I would like it to become more holistic and, generally, the public to understand much more about what we mean. I'd like public health to be doing more of the public inspiration stuff and culture change and thinking more creatively about the skills that it needs actually ... If it's

going to be really improving people's health and reducing health inequalities, it needs to be much more creative and inclusive and open to learning.

For this interviewee and some of the others, public health objectives were likely to be far more achievable in a context in which the public were more aware of the factors shaping their health and were engaged with the aims and committed to the objectives of the public health system.

Many (although not all) of the interviewees therefore appeared to be more closely aligned with what has been termed the expert/evidence model of public health practice, rather than the leader/development model (Connelly and Emmel, 2003). The latter is associated with the role of public health advocates, interest groups and local communities in identifying and addressing threats to health. Greater involvement of disadvantaged communities is seen as key to addressing social exclusion and promoting regeneration. In this model, the role of the public health practitioner is described as facilitating collective action to achieve health. These conceptions of roles find a parallel in Elson's (2008) six models of joint DsPH, which include the expert and the community advocate and adviser. The models are not mutually exclusive and it is likely that DsPH will be required to perform some combination of them at different points in their careers.

Discussion and conclusion

On the journey that, in this and the two previous chapters, has taken us through the last few decades of the 20th century and the early years of the 21st century, what is striking is that many of the key issues facing public health remain so pertinent. They are reflected in the interviews reported in this book, and also in many of the policy debates around the purpose and nature of public health in modern society, a context in which the role of the 'expert' is questioned and where there is much greater emphasis on individual choice and personal responsibility for health. Indeed, if there is a defining theme running through the history of public health, it is what Berridge (2006: xxv) has termed a "preoccupation with occupational positioning". Perhaps of significance, too, is the fact that recent major reports from the Foresight group on obesity (Butland et al, 2007) and the Nuffield Council on Bioethics (2007) take a much broader cross-government, ecological approach to public health issues rather than one that is centred on the role of the NHS or on individual lifestyle change as represented by the government campaign to tackle obesity, 'Change4Life', which has been termed "a society-wide movement launching in January 2009 that will help every family in England eat well, move more and live longer by changing behaviour" (Department of Health, 2009b). In so doing, reports like Foresight's and the Nuffield Council's echo many of the classic reports on public health, notably the 1986 Ottawa Charter and WHO's *Health for All* initiative – a tradition upheld in the more recent report of the Commission on Social Determinants of Health (WHO, 2008a).

As we have shown, the history of public health in England is one marked by a community that remains fractured and seemingly at the mercy of successive NHS reorganisations, each of which has had the effect of further weakening the sector and preventing the development of effective and sustainable partnerships. Perhaps more importantly, and as noted near the start of this book, there remains what Lewis (1986) terms an absence of "philosophical underpinning" at the heart of public health, which is reflected in the health politics of 'prevention versus cure' in which 'cure' wins out most of the time in the competition for attention and resources. In the absence of a firm philosophical base to underpin its activities, key sections of the public health system have become preoccupied with the delivery of health care and have allowed others to tackle the wider determinants of health. Our study suggests that many of those working in public health within the NHS today continue to experience the considerable tension that Lewis highlighted in 1986 in "reconciling first their responsibility for the management of health services with that of analysing health problems and, second, their formal accountability to the NHS bureaucracy with their ethical accountability to their communities" (Lewis, 1986: 162). In many ways, the more interesting and innovative public health work has gone on outside the NHS in local government and among a few NGOs. There is nothing intrinsically wrong with this – indeed, it is entirely desirable and demonstrates that the public health system may well have a promising future. But, sadly, it is still the case that these efforts have tended on the whole to remain piecemeal and patchy and there remains a weakness in local government about its long-term commitment to a health agenda especially at a time of public spending cuts which will start to take effect from 2011. Conceivably the emergence of joint directors of public health, and perhaps other posts, at local level will begin to tackle this weakness and help strengthen capacity and capability. At the same time, while some issues, like partnership working, have a long and chequered history, others are of more recent origin and pose a significant challenge to traditional ways of thinking about and doing public health. For example, world class commissioning and its separation from providing services, together with growing diversity in the range of service providers and the extension of choice to users, are less familiar developments with which public health is rapidly having to come to terms. Many of these changes are resulting in a redefinition of what 'public' means and what constitutes the public realm. Traditional approaches and conceptions of the public interest appear to be changing. How far these changes will go, whether they will even survive and what their implications are for the future shape and direction of the public health function remains unclear.

But an issue that perhaps dominates the picture painted in this book, and is alluded to above, is the overriding tension between health care and health and the continuing imbalance between them, to which Wanless and others have pointed on numerous occasions. The NHS continues to dominate health policy, as it has done almost without interruption since its inception over 60 years ago, and, as a result, pulls the policy focus towards ill health and health care services. To put it bluntly, we have yet to put health before health care and prioritise health in decision making across the range of relevant policy areas.

The central contradiction running through health policy is nicely captured in the following quotation from Kimmo Leppo, Director-General of the Finnish Ministry of Social Affairs and Health:"one of the great paradoxes in the history of health policy is that, despite all the evidence and understanding that has accrued about determinants of health and the means available to tackle them, the national and international policy arenas are filled with something quite different" (quoted in Kickbusch, 2007: 157). Many of the views of our interviewees bear testimony to this paradox. Its impact is insidious as it corrupts any alternative conception of what a health system is or could be. Policy in what Kickbusch (2007) calls "health societies" still frames 'health' in terms of expenditure and consumption of health care services, and there is little differentiation between programmes that focus on health and those that focus on health care. Indeed, as Coote (2007: 138) claims:

> Health policy has been so thoroughly skewed towards illness and services that a visitor from outer space could be forgiven for assuming that the main role of government in this field is to fund and manage vast armies of doctors and nurses in hospitals up and down the country, all striving to repair sick bodies.

It is a dilemma that has plagued public health and an understanding of a public health system that is broader than health care services for at least a hundred years. There are some early encouraging, though still fragile, signs that through world class commissioning and other related developments the balance may be shifting. But whether these modest gains can survive the impact of savage cuts in public spending over the coming years, which will significantly affect what the NHS and local government among others can do, remains of significant concern. If history is any guide, public health will be an easy target for budget raids. It may be that some aspects of the system, notably health protection, will survive given the swine flu scare in 2009 and the expectation of future flu pandemics any time. But other areas of public health may become attractive for stripping out some of the growth in spending they have enjoyed over the past few years.

Political leadership is needed to bring about the required shift in emphasis in policy so that treatment services do not forever eclipse sustainable investment in public health measures. Indeed, the absence of political leadership compounds the IfG's criticism that cross-government working is woeful. It argues that "strengthening cross-departmentalism in Whitehall is essential to ensuring coherent policy and better service delivery" (Gash et al, 2008: 11).

The difficulties over the funding of public health are symptomatic of the dilemma of viewing the NHS as being at the centre of the public health system. Funding issues have plagued the progression of public health priorities for decades. The raiding of budgets in recent years, reported in the interviews, is therefore frustratingly familiar to those who have been involved in the field for some time. Arguments rage inconclusively around whether ring fencing is the answer or whether this is a sign of weakness and admission of defeat (Wilkinson, 2006). If public health were strong, so the argument runs, then why should ring fencing be necessary? The true measure of commitment to public health must surely be for mainstream budgets to apply to this sector as they do elsewhere in the acute sector. Why should public health be treated as a special case?

The view from Health England, the national reference group for health and wellbeing, is that public health may indeed be a special case and require incentives to ensure that more money is spent on preventive services. The dilemma facing public health, as perceived by the group, is that "the costs of most unhealthy activities impact in the future, whereas the benefits from them occur in the present" (Le Grand and Srivastava, 2009: 2). Following a review of possible incentives, they conclude that four score well on most criteria:

- matching grants to commissioners;
- matching grants to employers;
- direct payments or subsidies to individuals to discourage them from indulging in unhealthy activities such as smokiing while pregnant;
- taxes on unhealthy behaviours.

Libertarian paternalist policies, also known as 'nudge' policies following the work of Thaler and Sunstein (2008), and informed by the new behavioural economics (New Economics Foundation, 2005), are also deemed to be effective. These include adopting default positions such as removing all salt from all processed foods, which still leaves individuals with the choice of adding salt if they wish. Reducing portion sizes in restaurants would be another example.

However, none of these rather modest structural or policy changes is likely to happen or be sustainable without confronting some more fundamental concerns. Our review of the public health system over the past 30-plus years suggests that, unless there is some structured discourse around what public health is, what a public health system entails and why it has failed to meet expectations in the light of a mobilisation of bias in favour of health care services, then it is unlikely that major advances can be achieved. As we have sought to demonstrate, the 1986 Ottawa Charter, which has stood the test of time well, provides a framework within which such a debate may be conducted. As the International Union for Health Promotion and Education and the Canadian Consortium for Health Promotion Research have both proposed, "recommitment to the ideas of the Ottawa Charter and strengthening the conditions for effective health promotion are urgent matters. Health inequalities within and between nations are increasing worldwide" (Scriven, ed, 2007a: 3). The issue is revisited in the final report of the global Commission on Social Determinants of Health (WHO, 2008a). Building on this work in an English context, the Marmot review of health inequalities (Marmot Review, 2010) has set an ambitious agenda for public policy post-2010.

But, if the Marmot recommendations are to be successfully and fully implemented, those engaged in public health activity will need to become advocates for change. It is an issue mentioned by some of our interviewees, as well as by many observers and analysts over the years. Perhaps, therefore, the advocacy role of public health professionals requires strengthening. As Mackie and Sim (2007: 641) point out: "if we accept that being in public health requires us to be advocates for the health of the population we serve, then we should be adept in the art of rhetoric. We should be highly skilled persuaders of people, politicians and society as a whole to protect and promote the public health." In similar vein, Kickbusch (2004: 468) believes that public health must once again "become an art and a science", a discipline that is "fully engaged in the political and social arena" and mixes "wild passion" with reasoned analysis and sound evidence.

In the next, and final, chapter, we look ahead at some of the big policy challenges that seem likely to dominate much of the debate around the public's health in the remaining decades of the 21st century. These will confront any public health system regardless of the particular configuration of policies and structures.

SIX

Looking to the future

If we are to meet the daunting health challenges already known to exist as well as those that will, in all probability, arise in future (but which cannot yet be discerned), then those responsible for the health of the public need to raise their game and their sights well above what Wanless et al (2007: xxvi) call "piecemeal, often modest initiatives".

What are the 21st-century health challenges confronting us? Collectively, as Marmot and Bell (2009), among others, have pointed out, we face several global problems in need of solutions. Two in particular stand out and most of the others are linked to them, in one way or another:

- the problem of climate change and environmental degradation and their consequences for, and impact on, health;
- growing inequalities within countries, combined with huge global inequities in social conditions and health.

A third challenge, which is not considered in detail here, concerns infectious diseases and pandemics. To some extent, these are driven by the other two challenges, particularly when it comes to their global diffusion. Although these three challenges can be regarded as separate and distinct, they are closely interconnected and no country, regardless of its wealth, will be immune from, or unaffected by, them. For example, the risk of pandemics arising from new strains of flu – the most recent example of which concerns swine flu, which originated in Mexico but spread rapidly to the US and to countries in Europe, including the UK – is increased as a result of greater mobility, global interdependence, international air travel and cheap flights. Even climate change may play a part in the transmission of infectious diseases.

Whether these factors will continue to grow and have such a profound effect on disease and its transmission will depend to some extent on what happens to our collective response to the environment, climate change and peak oil. It may be that the volume of international travel could be a victim of the depletion of fossil fuels. At the same time, the growing evidence of health inequalities within and between countries could well be a factor in the spread of infectious diseases. Furthermore, many of the people already living in difficult circumstances are those most at risk of experiencing poor health and are also likely to suffer more from the adverse effects of climate change and related problems.

The remainder of this chapter considers each of the two major primary challenges noted above and their impact on public health.

Climate change, environmental degradation and health

Perhaps the most complex challenge facing public health concerns climate change and environmental degradation. As Kickbusch puts it, there is remarkable congruence between the state of public health and the state of the environment, although their interdependence has perhaps not caught the public mood to the extent necessary to bring about an urgent political commitment to change (Kickbusch, 2008). Both are in crisis and, on their present respective trajectories, "run counter to the notion of sustainable wellbeing" (Kickbusch, 2008: 6). Both focus on the ways of living that have evolved in our societies, many of which are major contributors to the "diseases of comfort" that are responsible for growing levels of chronic illness and are likely to be major causes of death in the 21st and 22nd centuries (Choi et al, 2005). And both indicate that:"significant changes are required at the level of policy and of society" (Kickbusch, 2008: 6). What remains to be fully understood in mainstream politics is how the adverse impact of our way of life on the environment is also counterproductive to our health and wellbeing. Since 2003, the UK Public Health Association (UKPHA) has taken the lead in pressing for a new concept of public health based on ecological principles in order to advance both the health of the people and the health of the planet (UKPHA, 2007). It is accepted that "there is an interdependence between health and sustainability which is neither fully recognised nor taken into account in policies and practice – a lack of shared meanings, understandings, and an absence of common vision, strategies, and programmes" (UKPHA, 2007: 16). In bringing together a range of public health and environmental organisations, the UKPHA's call for action sought to provide a single unifying framework to which people with disparate professional, disciplinary or sectoral perspectives could sign up. The need for action is urgent but is absent on the scale required. In particular, the UKPHA bemoaned the absence of effective leadership to offer clarity of purpose, commitment and drive.

Many clinicians and others believe climate change constitutes the biggest global threat to health in the 21st century, putting at risk the lives and wellbeing of billions of people through food and water shortages and extreme weather conditions (Haines et al, 2006; Stott and Godlee, 2006; WHO, 2006). Echoing the concerns of the UKPHA and others, they conclude that, despite mounting evidence, it is still not being taken seriously enough. The NHS has a particularly important part to play, given that it is the largest employer in Britain and a significant purchaser of products and services. While the Department of Health has set up a Sustainable Development Unit to provide advice and support to NHS managers and others, the NHS should be a leading voice in the debate and in finding solutions to reducing our carbon footprint. To that end, the report from *The Lancet* and University College London's Institute for Global Health Commission by Costello et al (2009) calls for "a new advocacy and public health movement" to bring together all those organisations and individuals with a role to play in adapting to the effects of climate change.

Unless we take action soon (and even then it may be too late), we may at best simply be limiting the damage caused by climate change. In particular, heatwaves, such as occurred in Europe in 2003, which caused up to 70,000 'excess' deaths (Costello et al, 2009), will become more common, as will storms that cause flooding and structural damage. The result will be food and water shortages and no country will be immune from their impact. There is also a link between climate change and inequalities since, as noted, it will be the poorest people, wherever they are to be found across the world, who will be the worst affected and least protected.

Conversely, looking at the challenges both the public health and environmental agendas pose, it is possible to see numerous ways in which they can be linked to the mutual benefit of both so that health is improved and environmental degradation is arrested and possibly reversed. For example, if there was less use of vehicles, which led to more walking and cycling, then the health benefits that would accrue would include lower rates of injuries and deaths caused by road traffic accidents, lower stress levels, reduced obesity and lower risks from heart disease, lung disease and stroke. Such a health dividend in terms of improved wellbeing and greater social equity is not beyond our grasp, although it will be possible to achieve only if resistance from deeply entrenched interests is confronted and overcome. Advocates of such a shift, and who support a rebalancing of social and economic systems, view the global economic crisis as a once-in-a-lifetime opportunity to seize the initiative and adopt a new paradigm (Chan, 2009; Smith, 2009). But powerful forces, including most political leaders, appear to regard the crisis as a temporary blip, albeit a deep, lengthy and painful one, and believe (or hope) that at some point 'business as usual' will return (Cable,

2009). Perhaps a few lessons will have been learned from recent events so that in future there is less freedom for banks and tighter regulation of their operations. But, overall, there is a deep-seated conviction that the status quo ante will re-emerge, or be reinstated, in some form. Under such a scenario, the pressures and forces that contributed much to this crisis, which has swept through virtually every country's economy, will remain, possibly weakened but largely unchallenged.

If the opportunity presented by the economic crisis is lost, as seems all too likely, then we are likely to return to a situation in which tinkering with health care systems is a major focus of public policy activity in England, even though we (and, indeed, many managers and practitioners inside the system) are well aware that this is insufficient to improve health. The potential turning point in health policy, as advocated by Kickbusch (2008) and others (Chan, 2009; Smith, 2009), will remain elusive. Given what we know about the factors that create and sustain health (and perhaps the most persuasive recent review of the social failings of modern societies and the implications for health of the inequalities that they generate is that by Wilkinson and Pickett, 2009), as well as the evidence testifying to the rising rates of chronic disease, obesity, alcohol misuse and mental health problems, a new mindset in regard to health is urgently needed.

Hanlon and Carlisle (2008), while agreeing with this conclusion, go further and pose the question: are we facing a third revolution in human history? They believe we are and that the forces that prompted the first two great revolutions in human history – agriculture and industry – may well create the third revolution, which they argue is already upon us. These forces comprise population growth, resource pressures and chronic over-consumption by some societies (especially the US but others too). Such forces are undeniable features of the modern world. While a crisis can be creative and result in human adaptation to survive, it is also the case that adaptation is not a matter of choice for which people prepare but rather a reaction to an emergency that demands an immediate response. If this is the case, then the public health workforce will be faced with new challenges for which it may be ill-, or only partially, prepared. As Hanlon and Carlisle (2008: 360) put it: "if there is a role for public health professionals in facing new, 21st century challenges, then it will probably stem from the desire to prevent the adverse health consequences likely to result from continued adherence to the have-it-all, cornucopian mindset prevailing in contemporary Western societies". Public health practitioners will necessarily be in the frontline of action to prevent or ameliorate the harms that could flow from climate change and peak oil, as well as in terms of trying to realise the potential health dividend from achieving reduced levels of obesity, improved wellbeing and greater social equity.

To succeed in these endeavours, especially when governments still appear to fear being labelled 'nanny states' if they are seen to be telling people how to lead their lives, public health will have to confront those groups who, for whatever reason, are resistant to change, have vested interests, or oppose losing out on the allocation of resources that might otherwise go to public health. Such groups are likely to include large corporations who profit from the consumption of products that are contributing to contemporary health problems and climate change. For very different reasons, and as earlier chapters have shown, the history of public health in England suggests vigilance is also required to ensure resources intended for public health measures are not redirected to clinical and health service issues. Many of the latter kind of vested interests are, as earlier chapters have also shown, well to the fore within a country's health care system. There is also public reaction to contend with and while, for example, tobacco control measures have been gradually sanctioned by the majority of people, including many smokers, the same is not yet true for alcohol. As the Chief Medical Officer (CMO) for England acknowledges, "there is no stated national consensus that as a country we should substantially reduce overall alcohol consumption" (Department of Health, 2009c: 5). If evidence were needed of the complex interests at play, it can be found in the response to the CMO's plea, set out in his 2008 annual report, to raise the price of alcohol as a means of curbing binge drinking by ending the purchase of cheap alcohol from supermarkets (Department of Health, 2009c). No sooner had the suggestion been paraded in the media than politicians, from the Prime Minister down, had taken to the airwaves to denounce and distance themselves from the CMO's suggestion, on the grounds that the problem was more complex and that the proposed solution would unfairly penalise responsible drinkers. Needless to say, the drinks industry took a similar line, arguing that people had to be educated to drink sensibly and that merely raising the price of alcohol would do little to tackle the problem at source. Success in tobacco control has been in large part a result of public awareness about the impact of passive smoking. In contrast, the concept of 'passive drinking' is not yet recognised as a rationale for action although, in his annual report for 2008, the CMO believes its time may have come and that increasingly alcohol is seen as a problem not just for individuals but also for society as a whole. The passive effects, and associated collateral damage, include drink driving, family and marital breakdown, crime, domestic violence, problems at work and so on. But, because we do not yet know the total cost of passive drinking, it is easily ignored or dismissed as being of little consequence. However, like obesity, alcohol is a problem for everybody. Following the CMO's announcement, the British Medical Association, the National Institute for Health and Clinical Excellence, and the House of Commons Health Committee (2010) have come out in favour of a minimum price for a unit of alcohol, a move supported by the Scottish government but not by the UK government.

The immediacy of the reaction by the powerful drinks industry, combined with the Department of Health's willingness to include large 'junk food' manufacturers as partners in its more recent obesity initiative, 'Change4Life' (see Chapter Five), suggest that any lessons learnt with regard to the tobacco industry (for example, Neuman et al, 2002; Hastings and Angus, 2004; Diethelm and McKee, 2006; Mamudu et al, 2008) have not yet been extended to the many other areas of public health in which large, and often multinational, corporations play a key role (Freudenberg and Galea, 2007). For all 164 countries that have ratified the WHO's (2003) Framework Convention on Tobacco Control (FCTC), guidelines on Article 5.3 (which seeks to protect public health policies from tobacco industry interference) the tobacco industry can no longer be regarded as a stakeholder in the development of public health policies (WHO, 2008e). While many believe the situation with alcohol, food, oil and chemicals is more complex, companies in these sectors have already employed many of the same tactics as the tobacco industry in their efforts to avoid significant government regulation (Michaels and Monforton, 2005; Freudenburg et al, 2008; Michaels, 2008) and have sometimes collaborated directly with tobacco companies (Smith et al, 2010). This suggests it may make sense for public health advocates working in these different areas to learn from each other and to consider collaborating in efforts to ensure vested interests are not allowed to undermine the development of healthy public policies. As such, it may be worth considering whether Article 5.3 of the FCTC offers the opportunity for developing similar guidance to protect policies from alcohol, food, chemical and oil industry interference.

In order to embrace the challenge and tackle the vested interests that can become a barrier to change, and do so at a time when new resources are likely to be scarce or non-existent, it may be that we need to rethink the composition and purpose of the public health workforce and insist on public health becoming core business for those who may not naturally, or obviously, consider themselves to be engaged in public health work. If the health of nations is not primarily the result of modern medicine, as McKeown (1976) and many others since have argued, then we could perhaps do worse than follow the example of

Cuba, which has achieved 'first world' population health status at far less cost than is the case in developed high-income countries (Evans, 2008). The point is that, while medical care is 'powerful within limits', it cannot explain the major gradients in health within populations. As we have argued, and as many proponents of public health have insisted, income, education and other measures of social status are more significant determinants. But the Cuban health paradox is instructive. Despite poor economic performance, Cuba "has achieved and sustained health indices comparable to those in developed countries" (Spiegel and Yassi, 2004: 204). The country therefore refutes "the conventional assumption that generating wealth is a fundamental precondition for improving health" (Spiegel and Yassi, 2004: 204). So what is going on in Cuba? Are there lessons for others, at a time when wealth creation may not return to its former level (and perhaps should not do so, in the interests of sensible resource consumption)? Evans (2008: 30) argues that the Cuban experience "strongly supports the importance for population health of deliberate social action, of a very explicit focus not only on medical care but also on the non-medical determinants of health: education, nutrition, housing, employment and social cohesion".

But there is another factor and this is the active and wholesale embrace, rather than dismissal, of public health by the medical profession. Instead of regarding medical and non-medical determinants as competitive, which, as we have observed throughout this book, is a state of affairs that has arguably been to the detriment of the public health function and its development in England (and probably the UK as a whole), there is a case for regarding them as mutually reinforcing and as sharing the same primary goal, namely, securing better health outcomes for people and communities. Indeed, this division has contributed to public health's overall weakness and marginalisation, notwithstanding many examples of good practice. Moreover, it has led to the inefficient use of resources and risks making most health care systems unaffordable (Hunter, 2008). In contrast, and bucking the trend in spectacular fashion, Cuba has opted to address both medical and non-medical determinants of health with equal seriousness. As Evans (2008: 31) explains:

> ... primary care physician (and nurse) teams have responsibility for the health of geographically defined populations, not merely of those patients who come in the door. These teams are then linked to community – and higher-level political organisations that both hold them accountable for the health of their populations and provide

them with channels through which to influence the relevant non-medical determinants.

In Cuba, the health care system therefore works *with,* rather than in isolation from, the social determinants of health. It is an example of a truly integrated approach to health that has never been evident in the British NHS despite its enlightened and far-sighted founding principles with their emphasis on promoting health as well as treating ill health. It could be that such an arrangement constitutes a powerful lever for translating the evidence concerning the importance of social determinants into specific policies that are subsequently implemented.

Growing health inequalities and a widening health gap

The second challenge is one that we have already alluded to throughout the book. It concerns the widening health gap between social groups that is evident at all levels – that is, between countries, within countries, between regions within countries and even between small neighbourhoods within cities. Arguably, a concern with health inequalities on such a scale is a social justice issue rather than a public health one, but the fallout from a widening health gap nevertheless has major implications for public health as well as for health care and other public services (Wilkinson and Pickett, 2009). As many have argued, health inequalities are persistent, stubborn and difficult to change (for example, Davey Smith et al, 2001; Graham, 2007). It has often seemed easier to analyse their causes than to tackle them (Macintyre et al, 2001; Mackenbach, 2003). While overall levels of health have improved over the past decade or so, the gap between disadvantaged groups and areas and the rest of the population has remained and may even be widening. This is the conclusion of a review of developments in tackling health inequalities in England over the last ten years (Department of Health, 2009a). Current data (2005–07) show that it is no narrower than when the targets were first set in England, in 2001 (Department of Health, 2001a, 2001b). In his Foreword to the review, Marmot claims that, despite social and economic improvements, "persistent inequalities" remain "in income, educational achievement, literacy, child poverty, unemployment, local areas, anti-social behaviour and crime" (Department of Health, 2009a: 1). Part of the difficulty lies in the fact that, while health status is improving across all groups, it is improving at a faster rate in the most advantaged groups, resulting in the health inequalities gap continuing to widen. Moreover, health inequalities are not amenable to single or simple solutions but demand concerted action across government at all levels (Blackman et al, 2006). There also has to be a sustained focus on policy design and implementation, and avoidance of an endless stream of small-scale initiatives that all too often prove distracting and achieve little. Such initiatives can be designed to give the appearance of ministers taking action and doing something in response to a damning report or negative media coverage but they can so often lead to a dissipation of effort for little gain. A concern in the current economic climate must be that even the limited gains that have been achieved may prove short-lived unless the crisis has the effect of narrowing the income gap by preventing earnings at the top end of the scale from increasing as rapidly as they have in recent years.

The actions required to tackle the health inequalities that persist should be part of a broader coalition to promote social justice, with those working in public health in the vanguard of such a coalition. The Marmot review of health inequalities, conducted over one year (2009) at the request of the Prime Minister and the Health Secretary, affords a rare opportunity to progress the notion of a coalition as part of the new post-2010 agenda (Marmot Review, 2010). Apart from the attempt made to learn the lessons over the past ten years or so concerning the weaknesses in policy design and implementation, and the tendency endlessly to analyse the problems rather than act on them, the review's findings were launched in the midst of extremely difficult, if not hostile, economic conditions, which, when coupled with the environmental and sustainable development challenges noted above, put enormous pressure on a drive for social justice and narrowing the health gap. Keeping such issues alive and high on the policy agenda will be a considerable challenge in such circumstances, and will require political astuteness and well-developed skills at influencing policy, neither of which can be said to be currently in abundance within the public health community.

At the time of writing, and as noted earlier, we are in the midst of a global recession and financial crisis, the like of which the world has never before seen, at least in quite this configuration. There is little doubt that it will damage our health as well as our wealth but can it offer an opportunity to build a more equitable economic model? Although rich countries offer some protection to unemployed people through social safety nets, an economic downturn is still likely to bring with it deleterious consequences for health among those who are most disadvantaged (Marmot and Bell, 2009). It was ever thus. If work (and not just any work but employment that respects the rights of employees and does not worsen their health state) is not available to provide a route out of poverty (and associated ill health) then there will be negative consequences for the cognitive, emotional and physical development of children growing up in these circumstances and this will inevitably affect their long-term health and wellbeing. Whether the new global economic order that Marmot and Bell among others (for example, Chan, 2009) call for is a likely prospect remains uncertain. We are poised at a crossroads: do we strive to return to some version of the global economic growth trajectory that has led us to the situation in which we now find ourselves? Or do we take the long-term view and acknowledge that there can be no return to a model of economic growth that depends on the depletion of resources and a rise in greenhouse gases and that leads to inevitably obscene income inequalities?

The prospects for a new public health movement

The hope must be that the crisis that has befallen the global economy will provide an opportunity for radically rethinking the way we use scarce resources in our lives, including within health systems. This must include a reconsideration of the way we train expensive clinical staff, so that this incorporates an understanding of public health in its widest sense as being the core business of health care services as well as other services. Thinking 'outside the box', or out of the comfort zone of many groups, requires strong and committed leadership and a conviction that there has to be a better way, which can be achieved through using existing resources differently, rather than relying on injections of new resources that are simply not going to materialise in the near future, if at all. Yet, despite the plea not to lose the opportunity the crisis offers, it is hard to be optimistic about the chances of such new thinking taking root in mainstream policy making. Such thinking is far from absent but it is certainly not yet permeating or finding a strong voice in traditional political parties and governance arrangements. Rather, it is taking place on the fringes and is being driven by some left-of-centre think tanks and public health organisations like the UKPHA. These musings take us far beyond our focus on the public health system in England and its future prospects in the face of some complex and enduring problems, sometimes referred to as "wicked problems" (Rittel and Webber, 1973; Australian Public Service, 2007). However, the history of this system suggests that achieving any kind of radical change and overcoming long-standing problems is unlikely to be easy. This is exacerbated by the fact that most of the challenges facing public health are interconnected and developments elsewhere, particularly in the economic and/or environmental arenas, will unavoidably impact on the public health system. Indeed, they are already doing so. The positive, flip side of this interconnectedness is that, if achieved, a strong and confident public health system would be in a position to exert influence over what happens in these other domains. It is therefore surely in all of our interests, and those of future generations, that we succeed in making these connections.

When it comes to public health and its future in the midst of these twin challenges, there are those who believe that the present economic and political climate may be ripe for a revival of the spirit of Alma Ata. In 1978, this seminal Declaration established the goal of achieving health for all by the end of the century. Although that never happened, in part because of the harsh political and economic climate through most of the 1980s and 1990s brought about as a consequence of the rise of a neoliberal ideology, the initiative remains an inspiration and, as Baum (2007: 34) puts it: "a rallying call for progressive health workers and activists". While this far-sighted initiative did not foresee all of the current concerns facing public health, it remains "inspirational and visionary" (Baum, 2007: 35).

The prospects for a revival of what Alma Ata and *Health for All* stood for are encouraging, given the nature of the challenges facing public health in the 21st century. Although Alma Ata did not foresee the health impacts of climate change or the extent to which the marketisation of public policy (with its emphasis on 'consumers' and individuals rather than 'citizens' and communities) would occur, such developments would certainly be put under close scrutiny if it were to be updated. In any event, a revival of what Alma Ata stood for is evident in current assessments of health policy. Baum (2007) cites the WHO Commission on Social Determinants of Health as an example of a global initiative that echoes much of what appeared in the Alma Ata Declaration. And what Kickbusch (2008: 19) calls "the 'classic' determinants of health such as education, work, housing, transport and particularly equity... still have a major influence on health in the 21st century". Yet, paradoxically, and despite the evidence for an increase in attention to the underlying social determinants, most national public health policies concentrate on lifestyle factors. Sometimes, the broader public health aspects are included in general health policy but the importance of other sectors for health is perhaps less well developed. Nevertheless, there are signs, through initiatives such as Health in All Policies (HiAP), that this may be changing in some countries, with health equity appearing in the policies emerging from non-health sectors (Hogstedt et al, 2008). Even where this occurs, however, acting on commitments to improving and protecting health is a different matter and it is undeniable that further attention and effort are required on this front.

To a degree, the revival of the spirit of Alma Ata and other initiatives through the 1980s is also evident in the WHO European Region health charter, adopted in June 2008 in Tallinn, Estonia (WHO, 2008d). As we noted in Chapter One, the WHO view of health systems is one that encompasses "both personal and population services, as well as activities to influence the policies and actions of other sectors to address the social, environmental and economic determinants of health" (WHO, 2008d: 1). The charter is based on three central tenets: first, investing in health systems not only improves health and social wellbeing but also helps boost economic development (Figueras et al, 2008); second, it is unacceptable for people to become impoverished by ill health; and, third, health systems are as much about promoting health, preventing disease and ensuring health is considered in policies outside the health sector as they are about providing health care services. All of these sentiments are extremely worthy and laudable but what remains unclear, as it has done for some time, is whether the political motivation needed to act on such commitments can be found.

This chapter has described the key challenges and new forces, at least those we are presently aware of, which characterise the 21st century and may act to create or compromise health. Obesity may currently be viewed as the "symbolic disease of our global consumer society" and it will be the "test case for the health governance of the 21st century" since "it can only be resolved through great political commitment, willingness to innovate and social action at all levels of society" (Kickbusch, 2008: 22), but climate change and its potentially devastating impact on health could dwarf obesity in its significance and urgency. Whatever the challenge, having a strong vision and purpose will be essential but insufficient in the absence of political will and the emergence of a 'coalition of the willing' to bring about real and sustained change. That is the nature of the task that the public health community has faced for decades and seems likely to face well into the future. Unless or until it is successfully met, it is extremely unlikely that a strong or well-equipped public health system will emerge or be effective in meeting the challenges that lie ahead – and ones that may possibly be more complex and daunting than any so far witnessed.

NHS reorganisation – 1975–2009

The numerous reorganisations of the NHS since 1974 have each raised questions over the location and concentration of public health resources, the key responsibilities of public health professionals and their capacity to work effectively across health and local authorities, across regions and with primary care. The brief summary in this Appendix illustrates these points; diagrams are used to capture organisational snapshots within the various changes between 1974 and now.

Pre-1974 NHS: Medical Officer of Health

Up until 1974, the Medical Officer of Health (MOH) was based in local government, responsible for the health of the local population and the administration of community health services, including family planning, environmental health services, health visiting and health centres. The Health Education Council was formed in 1968 as a non-departmental body registered as a charity. The specialty of community medicine was formed in 1972, heralding its future role in the NHS. (Figure A.1 shows the pre-1974 NHS.)

Figure A1: The pre-1974 NHS

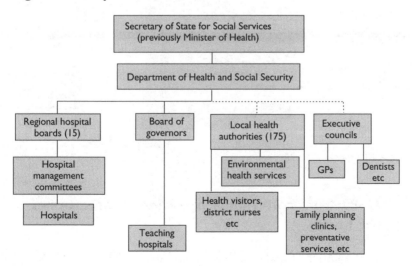

Source: Draper et al (1976)

1974–82: community physicians based in district health authorities

With the 1974 NHS reorganisation and the creation of regional, area and district health authorities and community health councils, MOsH were replaced by community physicians, located in the new district health authorities as district medical officers or specialists in community medicine, and in area health authorities (AHAs), where they became increasingly involved in management and administration. For the first time, personal health services and environmental health services were separated. The former executive councils were replaced by family practitioner committees; AHAs corresponded to the new local government boundaries (outside London); health education departments were accountable to AHAs. However, joint consultative committees were also formed across the NHS and local authorities to promote partnership working (Figure A.2 shows the 1974 NHS.)

Figure A2: The 1974 NHS

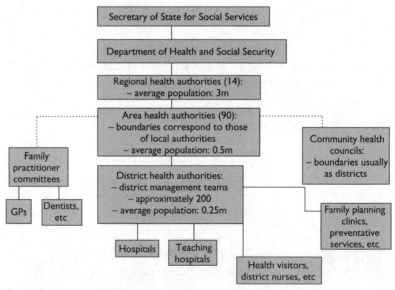

Source: Draper et al (1976)

1982–89: from community medicine to directors of public health

In 1982, the tier of management represented by AHAs was replaced by 192 restructured district health authorities (DHAs). Elected local government members formed part of their membership. In 1984, general management was introduced and, in 1986, the NHS Management Board was established. In 1989, this was reorganised into the NHS Policy Board and the NHS Management Executive. In 1988, the Department of Health split from the Department of Health and Social Security. It was recommended (Acheson, 1988) that each DHA appoint a Director of Public Health, that the term 'community medicine' be replaced by 'public health medicine', and that the annual report of the MoH be resurrected.

In 1985, family practitioner committees (FPCs) became autonomous bodies, accountable to the Secretary of State for Health. Collaboration across FPCs and DHAs, although essential for planning services, remained problematic. The Health Education Authority was established as a special health authority within the NHS in 1987, now directly accountable to the Secretary of State for Health.

1989–97: purchasers and providers

Following the White Paper, *Working for Patients* (1989) (Secretaries of State for Health, Scotland, Wales and Northern Ireland, 1989), which established the purchaser–provider split in the NHS, the internal market was introduced in 1991 and, from 1991 to 1995, stand-alone NHS trusts were created. DHAs became health authorities (1991) with business-style management boards and responsibility for commissioning services and assessing health needs. DsPH became involved in purchasing. Also in 1991, FPCs became family health service authorities (FHSAs), coterminous with the health authorities. In 1996, regional health authorities were reorganised and reduced in number from 14 to eight. They were known as regional offices of the NHS Executive. In 1994, nine government offices were set up, one for each region in England, although there was a lack of coterminosity between the regional offices of the NHS Executive and government offices.

Health authorities (HAs) took on a number of public health functions previously undertaken by the regional offices (for example, surveillance). While each regional office had a regional director of public health, they no longer published annual reports.

In 1996, FHSA responsibilities were merged into those of health authorities. Responsibility for health strategies rested with the HAs. It was argued that a fragmentation of purchasers and providers would make coordinated planning more difficult (Figure A.3 shows the 1996 NHS).

Figure A3: The 1996 NHS

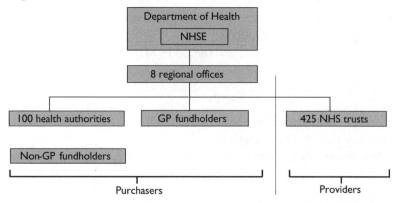

1997–2009: from health authorities to primary care trusts

In 1999, following publication of the 1997 White Paper *The New NHS: Modern Dependable* (Secretary of State for Health, 1997), 481 primary care groups (later primary care trusts, PCTs) were established. HAs were tasked with producing three-year health improvement programmes, in collaboration with primary care groups and local authorities, drawing on the Director of Public Health's Annual Public Health Report and in the context of the public health strategy, *Saving Lives: Our Healthier Nation*, published in 1999 (Secretary of State for Health, 1999). In 2000, the first wave of PCTs was established and, in 2001, *Shifting the Balance of Power* (Department of Health, 2001d) announced that 302 PCTs and 28 strategic health authorities (SHAs) would replace the 95 health authorities and the nine regional offices of the NHS Executive; this was completed in 2002. Regional health authorities were abolished and regional directors of public health were based at government offices while both SHAs and PCTs had directors of public health. In 2003, the four Regional Directorates for Health and Social Care were abolished. The Health Development Agency was established as a special health authority in 2000 and the Health Protection Agency was established as a special health authority in 2003. (Figure A.4 shows the 2004 NHS.)

Figure A4: The 2004 NHS

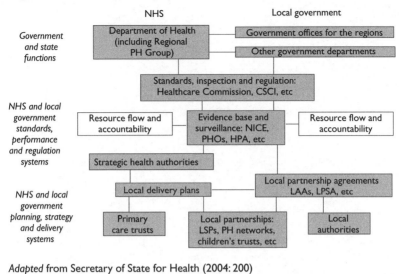

Adapted from Secretary of State for Health (2004: 200)

2005–present: more reconfiguration

Following publication of *Commissioning a Patient-led NHS* in 2005 (Department of Health, 2005c), strategic health authorities were reconfigured (in 2006) to match the boundaries of government offices, reducing their number from 28 to ten. Primary care trusts were reduced in number from 303 to 152 (mirroring the number of the former district health authorities) and the majority were designed to be coterminous with local authorities. In 2006, a single director of public health post was established at regional level, combining the remits of regional director of public health, strategic health authority director of public health and medical director posts. At PCT level, encouragement was given to making the DPH a joint post between the NHS and local government and, by early 2007, most of the new DPH appointments were joint, although the term 'joint' could mean very different things in different health communities. The Health Protection Agency was established as a non-departmental public body in 2005, accountable through the Department of Health. Also in 2005, the Health Development Agency was subsumed within the National Institute for Clinical Excellence, which was renamed the National Institute for Health and Clinical Excellence while retaining the acronym, NICE.

References

Abbott, S. and Killoran, A. (2005) *Mapping public health networks*, London: HDA.

Abbott, S., Petchey, R., Kessel, A. and Killoran, A. (2005) 'What sort of networks are public health networks?', *Public Health*, 120(6), 551-6.

Acheson, D. (1988) *Public health in England. The report of the committee of inquiry into the future development of the public health function*, London: HMSO.

Acheson, D.C. (1998) *Independent inquiry into inequalities in health*, London: The Stationery Office.

Alderslade, R. and Hunter, D.J. (1994) 'Commissioning and public health', *Journal of Management and Medicine*, 8(6), 20-31.

Alimo-Metcalfe, B. (2008) *Building leadership capacity through engaging leadership*, Selected reports from the 12th World HR Congress, London.

Ashton, J. (1984) *Health in Mersey – a review*, Liverpool: Department of Community Health, Liverpool University Medical School.

Ashton, J. (1988) 'Acheson: a missed opportunity for the new public health', *British Medical Journal (Clin Res Ed)*, 296(6617), 231-2.

Ashton, J. and Seymour, H. (1988) *The new public health*, Milton Keynes: Open University Press.

Audit Commission (2009) *Means to an end: Joint financing across health and social care*, Health National Report, London: Audit Commision.

Audit Commission and Healthcare Commission (2008) *Is the treatment working? Progress with the NHS system reform programme*, Health National Report, London: Audit Commission.

Audit Commission, Care Quality Commission, HM Inspectorate of Constabulary, HM Inspectorate of Prisons, HM Inspectorate of Probation and Ofsted (2009) *Comprehensive Area Assessment: A guide to the new framework*, London: Audit Commission.

Australian Public Service (2007) *Tackling wicked problems: A public policy perspective*, Canberra: Commonwealth of Australia.

Baggott, R. (2000) *Public health: Policy and politics*, Basingstoke, Macmillan.

Baggott, R. (2005) 'From sickness to health? Public health in England', *Public Money and Management*, August, 229-36.

Barton, H. and Grant, M. (2006) 'A health map for the local human habitat', *The Journal of the Royal Society for the Promotion of Health*, 126(6), 252-3.

Barts and City University London (2003) *Capacity and development needs of primary care trust and strategic health authority specialists in public health*, London: Barts and City University London.

Bauld, L., Judge, K., Barnes, M., Mackenzie, M. and Sullivan, H. (2005) 'Promoting social change: the experience of Health Action Zones in England', *Journal of Social Policy*, 34: 427-45.

Bauld, L., Judge, K., Lawson, L., Mackenzie, M., Mackinnon, J. and Truman, J. (2001) *Health Action Zones in transition: Progress in 2000*, Glasgow: Health Promotion Policy Unit, University of Glasgow.

Baum, F. (2007) 'Health for all now! Reviving the spirit of Alma Ata in the twenty-first century: an introduction to the Alma Ata Declaration', *Social Medicine*, 2(1), 34-41.

Beaglehole, R., Bonita, R., Horton, R., Adams, O. and McKee, M. (2004) 'Public health in the new era: improving health through collective action', *The Lancet*, 363(9426), 2084-6.

Benzeval, M. (2003) *The final report of the tackling inequalities in health module*, London: Queen Mary, University of London.

Berridge, V. (1999) *Health and society in Britain since 1939*, Cambridge: Cambridge University Press.

Berridge, V. (2000) 'History in public health: who needs it?', *The Lancet*, 356(9245), 1923-5.

Berridge, V. (2006) 'Introduction', in V. Berridge, D.A. Christie and E.M. Tansey (eds) *Public health in the 1980s and 1990s: Decline and rise? The transcript of a witness seminar, 12 October 2004*, London: Wellcome Trust Centre for the History of Medicine at UCL.

Berridge, V. and Blume, S. (eds) (2003) *Poor health: Social inequality before and after the Black Report*, London: Frank Cass.

Berridge, V., Christie, D.A. and Tansey, E.M. (eds) (2006) *Public health in the 1980s and 1990s: Decline and rise? The transcript of a witness seminar, 12 October 2004*, London: Wellcome Trust Centre for the History of Medicine at UCL.

Blackman, T. (2006) *Placing health: Neighbourhood renewal, health improvement and complexity*, Bristol: The Policy Press.

Blackman, T., Elliott, E., Greene, A., Harrington, B., Hunter, D.J., Marks, L., McKee, L. and Williams, G. (2006) 'Performance assessment and wicked problems: the case of health inequalities', *Public Policy and Administration*, 21(2), 66-80.

Blaxter, M. (1997) 'Whose fault is it? People's own conceptions of the reasons for health inequalities', *Social Science and Medicine*, 44(6), 747-56.

Blears, H. (2002) 'The challenges facing public health', Speech to Annual Scientific Conference of Faculty of Public Health Medicine, 27 June, London: Department of Health.

Bonner, L. (2003) 'Using theory-based evaluation to build evidence-based health and social care policy and practice', *Critical Public Health*, 13(1), 77-92.

Brackenridge,G.R.(1981) 'Community medicine: a revised prescription', *Public Health*, 95(3), 139-42.

Brown, G. (2008) 'Speech on the National Health Service', 7 January (www.pm.gov.uk).

Brown, J. (2002) *Public health workforce scoping study for the North East and Yorkshire and Humber. A report for the Health Development Agency.*

Brown, J.S. and Learmonth, A. (2005) 'Mind the gap: developing the public health workforce in the North East and Yorkshire and Humber regions: a scoping stakeholder study', *Public Health*, 119(1), 32-8.

Burke, S., Meyrick, J. and Speller,V. (2001) *Public health skills audit 2001: Research report*, London: Health Development Agency.

Burnham, A. (2009) 'Embrace new era of redesign to take NHS from good to great', *Health Service Journal*, 119(6180), 12-13.

Burton, P. (2001) 'Wading through the swampy lowlands: in search of firmer ground in understanding public policymaking', *Policy & Politics*, 29(2), 209-17.

Burton, S. and Diaz de Leon, D. (2002) 'An evaluation of benefits advice in primary care: Camden and Islington Health Action Zone', in L. Bauld and K. Judge (eds) *Learning from Health Action Zones*, Chichester: Aeneas Press, pp 241-50.

Buse, K. and Lee, K. (2005) *Business and global health governance*, Discussion paper no 5 (www.lshtm.ac.uk/cgch/Discussion%20Paper%205_Business%20and%20Global%20Health%20Governance_1.pdf).

Butland, B., Jebb, S., Kopelman, P., McPherson, K., Thomas, S., Mardell, J. and Parry, V. (2007) *Tackling obesities: Future choices – Project report*, Commissioned by the UK Government's Foresight Programme, Government Office for Science, London: Department of Innovation, Universities and Skills.

Byrne, D. (1998) *Complexity theory and the social sciences*, London: Routledge.

Cabinet Office (1999) *Modernising government*, London: The Stationery Office.

Cabinet Office (2007) *Capability review of the Department of Health*, London: Cabinet Office.

Cabinet Office (2009) *Capability reviews: Department of Health: Progress and next steps*, London: Cabinet Office.

Cable, V. (2009) *The storm: The world economic crisis and what it means*, London: Atlantic Books.

Calman, K.C. (1998) *The potential for health*, Oxford: Oxford University Press.

Chan, M. (2009) *Impact of financial crisis on health: A truly global solution is needed*, Geneva: WHO (www.who.int/mediacentre/news/statements/2009/financial_crisis_20090401/en/index.html).

Chapman, J. (2004) *System failure: Why governments must learn to think differently* (2nd edn), London: Demos.

Chapman, J., Abbott, S. and Carter, Y.H. (2005) 'Developing a speciality: regearing the specialist public health workforce', *Public Health*, 119(3), 167-73.

Chapman, J., Shaw, S., Congdon, P., Carter, Y.H., Abbott, S. and Petchey, R. (2005) 'Specialist public health capacity in England: working in the new primary care organizations', *Public Health*, 119(1), 22-31.

Choi, B.C.K., Hunter, D.J., Tsou, W. and Sainsbury, P. (2005) 'Diseases of comfort: primary cause of death in the 22nd century', *Journal of Epidemiology & Community Health*, 59(12): 1030-4.

Connelly, J. and Emmel, N. (2003) 'Preventing disease or helping the struggle for emancipation: does professional public health have a future?', *Policy & Politics*, 31(4), 565-76.

Connelly, J., McAveary, M. and Griffiths, S. (2005) 'National survey of working life in public health after "Shifting the Balance of Power": results of first survey', *Public Health*, 119(12):1133-7.

Coote, A. (2007) 'Labour's health policy – the cart before the horse?', *Soundings*, 35: 137-47.

Corrigan, P. (2007) 'New social democratic politics of public health in England today', in S. Griffiths and D.J. Hunter (eds) *New perspectives in public health* (2nd edn), Oxford: Radcliffe Publishing.

Corrigan, P. (2009) 'Why Burnham is wrong to rip up the competition rulebook', *Health Service Journal*, 119(6180), 14-15.

Cosford, P., O'Mahony, M., Angell, E., Bickler, G., Crawshaw, S., Glencross, J., Horsley, S.S., McCloskey, B., Puleston, R., Seare, N. and Tobin, M.D. (2006) 'Public health professionals' perceptions toward provision of health protection in England: a survey of expectations of Primary Care Trusts and Health Protection Units in the delivery of health protection', *BMC Public Health*, 6: 297.

Costello, A., Abbas, M., Allen, A. et al (2009) 'Managing the health effects of climate change', *The Lancet*, 373(9676): 1693-733, Doi: 10.1016/50140-6736(09)60935-1 (www.thelancet.com).

Cross-Government Obesity Unit, Department of Health and Department for Children, Schools and Families (2008) *Healthy weight, healthy lives: A cross-government strategy for England*, London: HM Government.

Crowley, P. and Hunter, D.J. (2005) 'Putting the public back into public health', *Journal of Epidemiology and Community Health*, 59(4), 265-7.

Dahlgren, G. and Whitehead, M. (1991) *Policies and strategies to promote social equity in health*, Stockholm: Institute of Futures Studies.

Davenport, C., Mathers, J. and Parry, J. (2006) 'Use of health impact assessment in incorporating health considerations in decision making', *Journal of Epidemiology and Community Health*, 60(3), 196–201.

Davey Smith, G., Dorling, D. and Shaw, M. (eds) (2001) *Poverty, inequality and health in Britain: 1800-2000 – A reader*, Bristol: The Policy Press.

Davis, P. and Lin, V. (2004) 'Public health in Australia and New Zealand', in R. Beaglehole (ed) *Global public health: A new era*, Oxford: Oxford University Press.

Department for Business, Enterprise and Regulatory Reform (undated) *Impact assessment guidance* (www.berr.gov.uk/files/file44544.pdf).

Department of Community Health (1986) 'The future development of the public health function and of community medicine (submission of evidence to the DHSS Committee of Inquiry)', London: LSHTM (unpublished).

Department of Health (1997) *The new NHS: Modern, dependable*, Cm 3807, London: The Stationery Office.

Department of Health (1998a) *The health of the nation – A policy assessed*, London: The Stationery Office.

Department of Health (1998b) *Chief Medical Officer's Project to Strengthen the Public Health Function in England: A report of emerging findings*, London: Department of Health.

Department of Health (1998c) *A first class service: Quality in the new NHS*, London: Department of Health.

Department of Health (2000) *NHS plan: A plan for investment, a plan for reform*, London: Department of Health.

Department of Health (2001a) *From vision to reality*, London: Department of Health.

Department of Health (2001b) *Health Secretary announces new plans to improve health in poorest areas*, London: Department of Health.

Department of Health (2001c) *The report of the Chief Medical Officer's Project to Strengthen the Public Health Function*, London: Department of Health.

Department of Health (2001d) *Shifting the balance of power within the NHS: Securing delivery*, London: Department of Health.

Department of Health (2002) *Getting ahead of the curve: A strategy for combating infectious diseases*, London: Department of Health.

Department of Health (2003a) *Tackling health inequalities: A programme for action*, London: Department of Health.

Department of Health (2003b) *Choice, responsiveness and equity in the NHS and social care: A national consultation*, London: Department of Health.

Department of Health (2004) *Agenda for change: Proposed agreement on modern pay and conditions for NHS staff*, London: Department of Health.

Department of Health (2005a) *Delivering choosing health: Making healthier choices easier*, London: Department of Health.

Department of Health (2005b) *New task force to help voluntary sector get involved in health and social care*, Press release, London: Department of Health.

Department of Health (2005c) *Commissioning a patient-led NHS* Cm 6268, London: Department of Health

Department of Health (2006) *Annual report 2005: The Chief Medical Officer on the state of public health*, London: Department of Health.

Department of Health (2007a) *What is public health?* (www.dh.gov.uk)

Department of Health (2007b) *2006 annual report of the Chief Medical Officer: On the state of public health*, London: Department of Health.

Department of Health (2007c) *Development plan*, London: Department of Health.

Department of Health (2007d) *Commissioning framework for health and well-being*, London: Department of Health.

Department of Health (2007e) *World class commissioning: Vision*, London: Department of Health.

Department of Health (2008a) *High quality care for all: NHS next stage review final report*, Cm 7432, London: Department of Health.

Department of Health (2008b) *World class commissioning: Commissioning assurance handbook*, London: Department of Health.

Department of Health (2009a) *Tackling health inequalities: 10 years on – A review of developments in tackling health inequalities in England in the last 10 years*, London: Department of Health.

Department of Health (2009b) *Be active, be healthy: A plan for getting the nation moving*, London: Department of Health.

Department of Health (2009c) *150 years of the Annual Report of the Cheif Medical Officer: On the state of public health 2008*, London: Department of Health.

Department of Health and Social Security (1980) *Inequalities in health: Report of a research working group*, The Black Report, London: Department of Health and Social Security.

Department of Health and Social Security (1986) *Report of the committee of inquiry into an outbreak of food poisoning at Stanley Royd Hospital*, Cm 9716, London: HMSO.

Department of Health and the Welsh Assembly Government (2004) *Shaping the future of health promotion in the NHS*, London: Department of Health.

Diethelm, P. and McKee, M. (2006) *Lifting the smokescreen: Tobacco industry strategy to defeat smoke free policies and legislation*, Brussels: European Respiratory Society and Institut National du Cancer (INCa).

Donaldson, R.J. and Hall, D.J. (1979) 'The work of the community physician in England', *Community Medicine*, 1(1), 52-68.

Dorling, D., Shaw, M. and Davey Smith, G. (2007) 'Inequalities in mortality rates under New Labour', in E. Dowler and N. Spencer (eds) *Challenging health inequalities: From Acheson to 'Choosing Health'*, Bristol: The Policy Press.

Dowler, E. and Spencer, N. (eds) (2007) *Challenging health inequalities: From Acheson to 'Choosing Health'*, Bristol: The Policy Press.

Draper, P., Grenholm, G. and Best, G. (1976) 'The organization of health care: a critical view of the 1974 reorganization of the National Health Service', in D. Tuckett (ed) *An introduction to medical sociology*, London: Tavistock Publications.

Duggan, M. (2001) *Healthy living: The role of modern local authorities in creating healthy communities*, Birmingham: SOLACE.

Editorial (1981) 'The Medical Officer of Environmental Health', *Public Health: The Journal of the Society of Community Medicine*, 95(5), 247-9.

Editorial (2009) 'Change4Life brought to you by PepsiCo (and others)', *The Lancet*, 373 (9658), 96.

Ellis, T. (2005) *Regional public health systems event workshop*, Stockport: North West Strategic Health Authorities and Government Office North West.

Elson, T. (1999) 'Public health and local government', in S. Griffiths and D.J. Hunter (eds) *Perspectives in public health*, Oxford: Radcliffe Medical Press.

Elson, T. (2004) 'Why public health must become a core part of council agendas', in K. Skinner (ed) *Community leadership and public health: The role of local authorities*, London: The Smith Institute.

Elson, T. (2007) 'Local government and the health improvement agenda', in S. Griffiths and D.J. Hunter (eds) *New perspectives in public health* (2nd edn), Oxford: Radcliffe Publishing.

Elson, T. (2008) 'Joint Director of Public Health appointments – 6 models of practice', in D.J. Hunter (ed) *Perspectives on joint Director of Public Health appointments*, London: Improvement & Development Agency.

Evans, D. (2003) '"Taking public health out of the ghetto": the policy and practice of multi-disciplinary public health in the United Kingdom', *Social Science and Medicine*, 57(6), 959-67.

Evans, D. and Dowling, S. (2002) 'Developing a multi-disciplinary public health specialist workforce: training implications of current UK policy', *Journal of Epidemiology and Community Health*, 56(10), 744-7.

Evans, D. and Knight, T. (2006) *'There was no plan!': The origins and development of multi-disciplinary public health in the UK*, Witness seminar, Bristol: University of the West of England.

Evans, R.G. (2008) 'Thomas McKeown, meet Fidel Castro: physicians, population health and the Cuban paradox', *Healthcare Policy*, 3(4), 21-32.

Faculty of Public Health (2006) *Specimen job description for directors of public health*, London: Faculty of Public Health.

Faculty of Public Health (2007) *What is public health?*, London: Faculty of Public Health (www.fphm.org.uk/about_faculty/what_public_health/default.asp).

Fahey, D.K., Carson, E.R., Cramp, D.G. and Muir Gray, J.A. (2003) 'User requirements and understanding of public health networks in England', *Journal of Epidemiology and Community Health*, 57(12), 938-44.

Farrell, C. (2004) *Patient and public involvement in health: The evidence for policy implementation*, London: Department of Health.

Figueras, J., McKee, M., Lessof, S., Duran, A. and Menabde, N. (2008) *Health systems, health and wealth: Assessing the case for investing in health systems*, Copenhagen: WHO.

Fotaki, M. (2006) 'Choice is yours: a psychodynamic exploration of health policymaking and its consequences for the English NHS', *Human Relations*, 59(12), 1711-44.

Fotaki, M. (2007) 'Can Directors of Public Health implement the new public health agenda in primary care? A case study of primary care trusts in the North West of England', *Policy & Politics* 33(2), 311-335.

Fotaki, M., Boyd, A., Smith, L., McDonald, R., Edwards, A., Elwyn, G., Roland, M. and Scheaff, R. (2006) *Patient choice and the organisation and delivery of health services: Scoping review*, report for the NCCSDO, Manchester: University of Manchester, Centre for Public Policy and Management.

Frenk, J. (1992) 'The new public health', in Pan American Health Organization *The crisis of public health: Reflections for debate*, Washington, DC: PAHO/WHO.

Freudenberg, N. and Galea, S. (2007) 'Corporate practices', in S. Galea (ed) *Macrosocial determinants of population health*, New York: Springer.

Freudenburg, W.R., Gramling, R. and Davidson, D.J. (2008) 'Scientific certainty argumentation methods (SCAMs): science and the politics of doubt', *Sociological Inquiry*, 78(1), 2-38.

Fry, J. (1968) *Profiles of disease*, Edinburgh: Livingstone.

Fulop, N. and Hunter, D.J. (1999) 'Editorial: saving lives or sustaining the public's health?' *British Medical Journal*, 319: 139-40.

Garrett, L. (2002) 'The collapse of global public health', *Health Matters*, 47: 8-10.

Gash, T., Hallsworth, M., Ismail, S. and Paun, A. (2008) *Performance art: enabling better management in the public services*, London: Institute for Government.

Gladwell, M. (2001) *The tipping point*, London: Abacus.

Glouberman, S. (2000) *Towards a new perspective on health and health policy: A synthesis document of the health network*, Ottawa: Canadian Policy Research Networks.

Goldenberg, M.J. (2005) 'On evidence and evidence-based medicine: Lessons from the philosophy of science', *Social Science and Medicine*, 62(11), 2621-2632.

Gorsky, M. (2007) 'Local leadership in public health: the role of the medical officer of health in Britain, 1872-1974', *Journal of Epidemiology and Community Health*, 61(6), 468-72.

Graham, H. (2007) *Unequal lives: Health and socioeconomic inequalities*, Maidenhead: Open University Press.

Gray, S. and Sandberg, E. (2006) *The specialist public health workforce in the UK, 2005 survey*, London: Faculty of Public Health.

Gray, S., Perlman, F. and Griffiths, S. (2005) 'A survey of the specialist public health workforce in the UK in 2003', *Public Health*, 119(10), 900-6.

Green, A., Ross, D. and Mirzoev, T. (2007) 'Primary care and England: the coming of age of Alma Ata?', *Health Policy*, 80(1), 11-31.

Greer, S. (2008) 'Devolution and divergence in UK health policies', *British Medical Journal*, 337: 2616.

Greer, S.L. (2005) 'The territorial bases of health policymaking in the UK after devolution', *Regional and Federal Studies* 15(4), 501-18.

Greer, S.L. (2007) 'Public health policy making in a disunited kingdom', in S. Griffiths and D.J. Hunter (ed) *New perspectives in public health* (2nd edn), Oxford: Radcliffe Publishing.

Greer, S.L. and Jarman, H. (2007) *The Department of Health and the civil service: From Whitehall to department of delivery to where?* London: The Nuffield Trust.

Greer, S.L. and Rowland, D. (2007) *Devolving policy, diverging values? The values of the United Kingdom's national health services*, London: The Nuffield Trust.

Griffiths, S. and Hunter, D.J. (eds) (2007) *New perspectives on public health* (2nd edn), Oxford: Radcliffe Publishing.

Griffiths, S., Jewell, T. and Donnelly, P. (2005) 'Public health in practice: the three domains of public health', *Public Health*, 119(10), 907-13.

Haines, A., Kovats, R.S., Campbell-Lendrum, D. and Corvalan, C. (2006) 'Climate change and human health: impacts, vulnerability, and mitigation', *The Lancet*, 367(9528), 2101-9.

Halliday, J. and Asthana, S. (2005) 'Policy at the margins: developing community capacity in a rural Health Action Zone', *Area*, 37: 180-8.

Ham, C. (2007) *Commissioning in the English NHS: The case for integration*, Nuffield Trust Series Report. London: The Nuffield Trust (www.nuffieldtrust.org.uk).

Hamlin, C. (2002) 'The history and development of public health in developed countries', in R. Detels, J. McEwan, R. Beaglehole and H. Tanaka (eds) *Oxford textbook of public health: The methods of public health* (4th edn), Oxford: Oxford University Press.

Hanlon, P. and Carlisle, S. (2008) 'Do we face a third revolution in human history? If so, how will public health respond?', *Journal of Public Health*, 30(4), 355-61.

Hannaway, C. (2008) 'The DPH role from a leadership perspective', in D.J. Hunter (ed) *Perspectives on joint Director of Public Health appointments*, London: Improvement & Development Agency.

Hannaway, C., Hunter, D.J. and Plsek, P. (2007) 'Developing leadership and management for health', in D.J. Hunter (ed) *Managing for health*, London: Routledge.

Harvey, S. and Judge, K. (1988) *Community physicians and community medicine: A survey report*, London: King's Fund Institute.

Hastings, G. and Angus, K. (2004) *The influence of the tobacco industry on European tobacco-control policy. Tobacco or health in the European Union – past, present and future*, Luxembourg: ASPECT Consortium, European Commission Directorate-General for Health and Consumer Protection.

Healthcare Commission (2004) *Standards for better health* (updated in 2006), London: Department of Health.

Healthcare Commission and Audit Commission (2008) *Are we choosing health? The impact of policy on the delivery of health improvement programmes and services*. London: Commission for Healthcare Audit and Inspection.

Health Service Journal (2009) News story, 23 August, p 5.

Hills, M. and McQueen, D. (eds) (2007) 'The Ottawa Charter for Health Promotion: a critical reflection', *Promotion and Education*, Supplement 2.

HM Treasury (2002) 2002 spending review, London: HM Treasury (www.hm-treasury.gov.uk/spend_sr02_psahealth.htm).

Hogstedt, C., Moberg, H., Lundgren, B. and Backhans, M. (eds) (2008) *Health for all? A critical analysis of public health policies in eight European countries*, Ostersund: Swedish National Institute of Public Health.

Holland, W.W. and Stewart, S. (1998) *Public health, the vision and the challenge*, London: Nuffield Trust.

Holman, J. (1992) 'Something old, something new: Perspectives on five 'new' public health movements', *Health Promotion Journal of Australia* 2: 4-11.

House of Commons Health Committee (2001a) *Public health: Second report session 2000/01*, volume I, report and proceedings of the committee (HC30), London: The Stationery Office.

House of Commons Health Committee (2001b) *Public health: Second report session 2000/01*, volume II, minutes of evidence and appendices (HC30-II), London: The Stationery Office.

House of Commons Health Committee (2009) *NHS next stage review. First report of session 2008–9,* volume I, report, together with formal minutes (HC53-1), London: The Stationery Office.

House of Commons Health Committee (2010) *Alcohol: First report of session 2009–10,* volume I, London: The Stationery Office.

House of Commons Public Administration Select Committee (2005) *Choice, voice and public services. Fourth report of session 2004–05. Volume 1*, London: The Stationery Office.

House of Lords (2006) *Lords Hansard text,* 7 December.

Hübel, M. and Hedin, A. (2003) 'Developing health impact assessment in the European Union', *Bulletin of the World Health Organization*, 81(6), 463-4.

Hughes, L. (2009) *Joint strategic needs assessment: Progress so far*, London: Improvement and Development Agency.

Hunter, D.J. (2003) *Public health policy*, Cambridge: Polity.

Hunter, D.J. (2005) 'Choosing or losing health?', *Journal of Epidemiology and Community Health*, 59(12), 1010-12.

Hunter, D.J. (2006) 'The National Health Service 1980-2005', *Public Money and Management*, 25(4), 209-12.

Hunter, D.J. (ed) (2007a) *Managing for health*, London: Routledge.

Hunter, D.J. (2007b) 'Exploring managing for health', in D.J. Hunter (ed) *Managing for health*, London: Routledge.

Hunter, D.J. (2008) *The health debate*, Bristol: The Policy Press.

Hunter, D.J. (ed) (2008) *Perspectives on joint Director of Public Health appointments*, London: Improvement & Development Agency.

Hunter, D.J. (2009) 'Response: The case against choice and competition', *Health Economics, Policy and Law*, 4(4), 489-501.

Hunter, D.J. and Marks, L. (2005) *Managing for health: What incentives exist for NHS managers to focus on wider health issues?*, London: King's Fund.

Hunter, D.J. and Sengupta, S. (2004) 'Building multi-disciplinary public health', *Critical Public Health*, 14(1), 1-5.

Hunter, D.J., Marks, L. and Smith, K. (2007) *The public health system in England: A scoping study*, London: NIHR SDO.

Institute of Medicine (1988) *The future of public health*, Washington, DC: The National Academies Press.

Institute of Medicine (2003) *The future of the public's health in the 21st century*, Washington, DC: The National Academies Press.

Jacobson, B., Smith, A. and Whitehead, M. (1991) *The nation's health: A strategy for the 1990s*, London: King Edward's Hospital Fund for London.

Jessop, E.G. (2002) 'Leading and managing public health networks', *Journal of Public Health Medicine*, 24(1), 1.

Jochelson, K. (2006) 'Nanny or steward? The role of government in public health', *Public Health*, 120(12), 1149-55.

Jong-wook, L. (2003) *Welcome speech, Second Consultation on Macroeconomics and Health*, Geneva: WHO.

Kane, B. (2002) 'Social capital, health and economy in South Yorkshire coalfield communities', in L. Bauld and K. Judge (eds) *Learning from Health Action Zones*, Chichester: Aeneas Press, pp 187-198.

Kawachi, I., Kennedy, B.P., Lochner, K. and Prothrow-Stith, D. (1997) 'Social capital, income inequality and mortality', *American Journal of Public Health*, 87(9), 1491-8.

Kelly, M., Morgan, A., Bonnefoy, J., Butt, J., Bergman, V., Mackenbach, J. et al (2007) *The social determinants of health: Developing an evidence base for political action,* Final report to World Health Organization Commission on the Social Determinants of Health (www.who.int/social_determinants/resources/mekn_report_10oct07.pdf).

Kelly, M.P. (2007) 'Evidence-based public health', in S. Griffiths and D.J. Hunter (eds) *New perspectives in public health* (2nd edn), Oxford: Radcliffe Publishing.

Kickbusch, I. (2004) 'The Leavell Lecture – the end of public health as we know it: constructing global health in the 21st century', *Public Health*, 118(7): 463-9.

Kickbusch, I. (2007) 'Health governance: the health society', in D. McQueen and I. Kickbusch (eds) *Health and modernity: The role of theory in health promotion*, New York: Springer.

Kickbusch, I. (2008) *Health societies: Addressing 21st century health challenges*, Adelaide: Government of South Australia.

Lalonde, M. (1974) *A new perspective on the health of Canadians*, Ottawa: Minister of Supply and Services.

Latter, S., Speller, V., Westwood, G. and Latchem, S. (2003) 'Education for public health capacity in the nursing workforce: findings from a review of education and practice issues', *Nurse Education Today*, 23(3), 211-18.

Le Grand, J. (2007a) *The other invisible hand: Delivering public services through choice and competition*, Princeton, NJ: Princeton University Press.

Le Grand, J. (2007b) 'The politics of choice and competition in public services', *The Political Quarterly*, 78(2), 207-13.

Le Grand, J. (2009) 'Debate: Choice and competition in publicly funded health care', *Health Economics Policy and Law* 4(4), 479-488.

Le Grand, J. and Hunter, D.J. (2006) 'Debate: choice and competition in the British National Health Service', *Eurohealth*, 12(1), 1-3.

Le Grand, J. and Srivastava, D. (2009) *Incentives for prevention*, Health England Report No. 3, London: Health England.

Lewis, J. (1986) *What price community medicine? The philosophy, practice and politics of public health since 1919*, Brighton: Wheatsheaf.

Lewis, J. (1987) 'From public health to community medicine: the wider context', in S. Farrow (ed) *The public health challenge*, London: Hutchinson.

Ling, T. (2002) 'Delivering joined-up government in the UK: Dimensions, issues and problems', *Public Administration*, 80(4), 615-42.

Local Government Association (2008) *Who's accountable for health?*, LGA Health Commission final report, London: LGA.

Local Government Association and UK Public Health Association (2000) *Joint response to the public health White Paper, 'Saving Lives: Our Healthier Nation'*, London: LGA.

Local Government Association, UKPHA and NHS Confederation (2004) *Releasing the potential for the public's health*, London: NHS Confederation.

Macintyre, S., Chalmers, I., Horton, R. and Smith, R. (2001) 'Using evidence to inform health policy: case study', *British Medical Journal*, 322(7280), 222-5.

Mackenbach, J.P. (2003) 'Tackling inequalities in health: the need for building a systematic evidence base', *Journal of Epidemiology and Community Health*, 57(3), 162.

Mackie, P. and Sim, F. (2007) 'Editorial: a question of rhetoric', *Public Health*, 121, 641-2.

Mallinson, S., Popay, J. and Kowarzik, U. (2006) 'Collaborative work in public health? Reflections on the experience of public health networks', *Critical Public Health*, 16(3), 259-65.

Mamudu, H.M., Hammond, R. and Glantz, S. (2008) 'Tobacco industry attempts to counter the World Bank report curbing the epidemic and obstruct the WHO framework convention on tobacco control', *Social Science and Medicine*, 67(11), 1690-9.

Mant, D. and Anderson, P. (1985) 'Community general practitioner', *The Lancet*, 326(8464),1114-7.

Marks, L. and Hunter, D.J. (2005) 'Moving upstream or muddying the waters? Incentives for managing for health', *Public Health*, 119: 974-80.

Marks, L. and Hunter, D.J. (2007) *Social enterprises and the NHS: Changing patterns of ownership and accountability*, London: UNISON.

Marmot Review, The (2010) *Fair society, healthy lives: Strategic review of health inequalities in England post-2010*, London: The Marmot Review.

Marmot, M.G. and Bell, R. (2009) 'How will the financial crisis affect health?', *British Medical Journal*, 338; doi:10.1136/bmj.b1314.

McAreavey, M.J., Alimo-Metcalfe, B. and Connelly, J. (2001) 'How do Directors of Public Health perceive leadership', *Journal of Management in Medicine*, 15(6), 446-62.

McKeown, T. (1976) *The role of medicine: Dream, mirage or nemesis*, London: Nuffield Provincial Hospitals Trust.

McPherson, K. (2000) 'Removing barriers to career development in public health', *British Medical Journal*, 320(7232), 448.

McPherson, K., Field, A. et al (1999) *Strengthening public health – proposals for national public health structures*, London: National Heart Forum.

McPherson, K., Taylor, S. and Coyle, E. (2001) 'For and against: public health does not need to be led by doctors', *British Medical Journal*, 322(7302), 1593-6.

Meads, G., Killoran, A., Ashcroft, J. and Comish, Y. (1999) *Mixing oil and water: How can primary care organisations improve health as well as deliver effective health care?*, London: Health Education Authority.

Michaels, D. (2008) *Doubt is their product – how industry's assault on science threatens your health*, New York: Oxford University Press.

Michaels, D. and Monforton, C. (2005) 'Manufacturing uncertainty: contested science and the protection of the public's health and environment', *American Journal of Public Health*, 95, S1, S39-S48.

Milburn, A. (2000) 'A healthier nation and a healthier economy: the contribution of a modern NHS', LSE Health Annual Lecture, 8 March, London.

Morgan, A. and Ziglio, E. (2007) 'Revitalising the evidence base for public health: an assets model', *Promotion & Education*, Supplement 2: 17-22 (available at: http://ped.sagepub.com/cgi/reprint/14/2_suppl/17).

Morris, J.N. (1969) 'Tomorrow's community physician', *The Lancet*, 294(7625) 2, 811–16.

Neuman, M., Bitton, A. and Glantz, S. (2002) 'Tobacco industry strategies for influencing European Community tobacco advertising legislation', *The Lancet*, 359(9314), 1323–30.

New Economics Foundation (2005) *Behavioural economics: Seven principles for policy-makers*. London: New Economics Foundation.

New South Wales Health Department (2001) *A framework for building capacity to improve health*, Gladesville: NSW Health Department.

Nicoll, A. (2007) 'Health protection and environmental public health in the UK and the rest of Europe', in S. Griffiths and D.J. Hunter (eds) *New perspectives in public health* (2nd edn), Oxford: Radcliffe Publishing.

Nuffield Council on Bioethics (2007) *Public health: ethical issues*, London: Nuffield Council on Bioethics.

Nutbeam, D. and Wise, M. (2002) 'Structures and strategies for public health intervention', in R. Detels, J. McEwen, R. Beaglehole and H. Tanaka (eds) *Oxford textbook of public health, vol 3: The practice of public health* (4th edn), Oxford: Oxford University Press.

Ollila, E., Lahtinen, E., Melkas, T., Wismar, M., Stahl, T. and Leppo, K. (2006) 'Towards a healthier future', in T. Stahl, M. Wismar, E. Ollila, E. Lahtinen and K. Leppo (eds) *Health in all policies: Prospects and credentials*, Helsinki: Finnish Ministry of Social Affairs and Health and European Observatiory on Health Systems and Policies.

Peckham, S. and Exworthy, M. (2003) *Primary care in the UK: Policy, organisation and management*, Basingstoke: Palgrave Macmillan.

Perkins, N., Smith, K.E., Hunter, D.J., Bambra, C. and Joyce, K.E. (2010) '"What counts is what works"? New Labour and partnerships in public health', *Policy & Politics*, 38(1): 101–17.

ph.com (2007) 'The public health future', September, the Newsletter of the Faculty of Public Health, www.fph.org.uk

Pickin, C., Popay, J., Staley, K., Bruce, N., Jones, C. and Gowman, N. (2002) 'Developing a model to enhance the capacity of statutory organisations to engage with lay communities', *Journal of Health Services Research and Policy*, 7(1), 34–42.

Pickles, H. (2004) 'Accountability for health protection in England: how this has been affected by the establishment of the Health Protection Agency', *Communicable Disease and Public Health*, 7(4), 241–4.

Pickles, W.N. (1929) *Epidemiology in a country practice*, Bristol: Wright.

Plsek, P. and Greenhalgh, T. (2001) 'The challenge of complexity in health care', *British Medical Journal*, 323(7313), 625–8.

Popay, J., Bennett, S., Thomas, C., Williams, G., Gatrell, A. and Bostock, L. (2003) 'Beyond "beer, fags, eggs and chips"? Exploring lay understandings of social inequalities in health', *Sociology of Health and Illness*, 25(1), 1-23.

Public Health Resource Unit and Skills for Health (2008) *Public health skills and career framework: Multidisciplinary/multi-agency/multi-professional*, Bristol: Skills for Health (www.publichealthdevelopment.org.uk/PH%20career%20framework%20Dec06).

Public Health Sciences Working Group (2004) *Health sciences: Challenges and opportunities*, London: Wellcome Trust.

Putnam, R.D. (2001) 'Social capital: measurement and consequences', in J.F. Helliwell (ed) *The contribution of human and social capital to sustained economic growth and well-being*, Ottawa: Human Resources Development, pp 117-35.

Rittel, H.W.J. and Webber, M.M. (1973) 'Dilemmas in a general theory of planning', *Policy Sciences*, 4(2), 155-69.

Ruhm, C. (2000) 'Are recessions good for your health?', *Quarterly Journal of Economics*, 115(2), 617-50.

Salay, R. and Lincoln, P. (2008) *The European Union and health impact assessments: Are they an unrecognised statutory obligation?*, London: National Heart Forum.

Saltman, R.B. and Ferroussier-Davis, O. (2000) 'The concept of stewardship in health policy', *Bulletin of the World Health Organisation* 78(6), 732-9.

Scally, G. and Womack, J. (2004) 'The importance of the past in public health', *Journal of Epidemiology and Community Health*, 58(9), 751-5.

Scottish Executive Health Department (1999) *Review of the public health function in Scotland*, Glossary (available at: http://www.scotland.gov.uk/library2/doc09/rphf-00.asp).

Scriven, A. (ed) (2007a) *Shaping the future of health promotion: Priorities for action*, Canada: IUPHE and CCHPR.

Scriven, A. (2007b) 'Healthy public policies: rhetoric or reality?', in A. Scriven and S. Garman (eds) *Public health: Social context and action*, Maidenhead: Open University Press.

Secretaries of State for Health, Wales, Scotland and Northern Ireland (1989) *Working for patients*, Cm 555, London: HMSO.

Secretary of State for Health (1992) *The health of the nation*, Cm 1986, London: HMSO.

Secretary of State for Health (1997) *The new NHS: Modern and dependable*, London: Department of Health.

Secretary of State for Health (1999) *Saving lives: Our healthier nation*, Cm 4386, London: The Stationery Office.

Secretary of State for Health (2004) *Choosing health: Making healthy choices easier*, Cm 6374, London: The Stationery Office.

Secretary of State for Health (2006) *Our health, our care, our say*, London: The Stationery Office.

Sihto, M., Ollila, E. and Koivusalo, M. (2006) 'Principles and challenges of Health in All Policies', in T. Stahl, M. Wismar, E. Ollila, E. Lahtinen and K. Leppo (eds) *Health in All Policies: Prospects and potentials*, Helsinki: Finnish Ministry of Social Affairs and Health and European Observatory on Health Systems and Policies.

Smith, K.E. (2009) 'A time for new beginnings', *Health Matters*, 75: 39.

Smith, K.E., Bambra, C., Joyce, K.E., Perkins, N., Hunter, D.J. and Blenkinsopp, E.A. (2009) 'Partners in health? A systematic review of the impact of organizational partnerships on public health outcomes in England between 1997 and 2008', *Journal of Public Health*, 31(2): 210-21.

Smith, K.E., Fooks, G., Collin, J., Weishaar, H., Mandal, S. and Gilmore, A. (2010) '"Working the system": British American Tobacco's influence on the European Union Treaty and its implications for policy: an analysis of internal tobacco industry documents', *PLoS Medicine* 7(1) (doi: www.plosmedicine.org/article/info:doi/10.1371/journal. pmed.1000202).

Smith, K.E., Fooks, G., Collin, J., Weishaar, H. and Gilmore, A. (in press) 'Is the increasing policy use of Impact Assessment in Europe likely to undermine efforts to achieve healthy public policy?', Accepted for publication in *Journal of Epidemiology and Community Health*, September 2009.

Somervaille, L. and Griffiths, R. (1995) *The training and career development needs of public health professionals: Report of postal survey and discussion workshops*, Birmingham: University of Birmingham.

Spiegel, J.M. and Yassi, A. (2004) 'Lessons from the margins of globalisation: appreciating the Cuba health paradox', *Journal of Public Health Policy*, 25(1), 96-121.

Ståhl, T. (2009) 'Is health recognised in the EU's policy process? An analysis of the European Commission's impact assessments', *European Journal of Public Health* (Advance online access at: http://eurpub. oxfordjournals.org/cgi/reprint/ckp082v1: 1-6).

Ståhl, T., Wismar, M., Ollila, E., Lahtinen, E. and Leppo, K. (eds) (2006) *Health in All pPolicies: Prospects and potentials*, Helsinki: Finnish Ministry of Social Affairs and Health and European Observatory on Health Systems and Policies (www.euro.who.int/document/E89260.pdf).

Stevens, S. (2004) 'Reform strategies for the English NHS', *Health Affairs*, 23(3), 37-44.

Stewart, G.T. (1987) 'Point of view: public health function', *The Lancet*, 329(8534), 695-6.

Stewart, M. (2007) 'Neighbourhood renewal and regeneration', in J. Orme, J. Powell, P. Taylor and M. Grey (eds) *Public health for the 21st century: New perspectives on policy, participation and practice* (2nd edn), Maidenhead: Open University Press.

Stone, D.H. (1987) 'Preventive care, community medicine and prevention: a convergence of needs', *Journal of the Royal College of General Practitioners*, 37(298), 218-20.

Stott, R. and Godlee, F. (2006) 'Editorial: what should we do about climate change? Health professionals need to act now, collectively and individually', *British Medical Journal*, 333(7576), 983-4.

Sullivan, H., Barnes, M. and Matka, E. (2002) 'Building collaborative capacity through theories of change', *Evaluation* 8: 205-226.

Sullivan, H., Judge, K. and Sewel, K. (2004) '"In the eye of the beholder": perceptions of local impact in English Health Action Zones', *Social Science and Medicine*, 59: 1603-12.

Sutherland, I. (1987) *Health education: Half a policy: The rise and fall of the Health Education Council*, Cambridge: NEC Publications.

Szreter, S. (2002) 'Rethinking McKeown: the relationship between public health and social change', *American Journal of Public Health*, 92(5), 722-5.

Taylor, P., Peckham, S. and Turton, P. (1998) *A public health model of primary care – from concept to reality*, Birmingham: Public Health Alliance.

Tenbensel, T. (2004) 'Does more evidence lead to better policy? The implications of explicit priority-setting in New Zealand's health policy for evidence-based policy', *Policy Studies* 25(3), 189-207.

Thaler, R.H. and Sunstein, C.R. (2008) *Nudge: Improving decisions about health, wealth, and happiness*, New York: Caravan Books.

Tilson, H. and Gebbie, K.M. (2004) 'The public health workforce', *Annual Review of Public Health*, 25: 341-56.

Tilson, H. and Berkowitz, B. (2006) 'The public health enterprise: examining our twenty-first-century policy challenges', *Health Affairs*, 25(4), 900-10.

Titmuss, R.M. (1965) 'The role of the family doctor today in the context of Britain's social services', *Lancet*, 1: 2.

Todd Commission (1968) *Report of the Royal Commission on Medical Education*, Cmnd 3569, London: HMSO.

Travis, P., Egger, D., Davies, P. and Mechbal, A. (2002) *Towards better stewardship: Concepts and critical issues* (WHO/EIP/DP 02.48), Geneva: WHO.

Tritter, J. and Lester, H. (2007) 'Health inequalities and user involvement', in E. Dowler and N. Spencer (eds) *Challenging health inequalities: From Acheson to 'Choosing Health'*, Bristol: The Policy Press.

Troop, P. (2007) 'The future of health protection', *ph.com*, September, 9 (www.fph.org.uk).

Tudor-Hart, J. (1988) *A new kind of doctor*, London: Merlin Press.

UKPHA (UK Public Health Association) (2007) *Climates and change: The urgent need to connect health and sustainable development*, London: UKPHA (www.ukpha.org.uk).

Unit for the Study of Health Policy (1979) *Rethinking community medicine*, London: Guy's Hospital Medical School.

Upward, J. (1998) *Rethinking public health: The first 10 years of the Public Health Alliance*, Birmingham: The Public Health Alliance.

Verweij, M. and Dawson, A. (2007) 'The meaning of "public" in "public health"', in A. Dawson and M. Verweij (eds) *Ethics, prevention and public health*, Oxford: Oxford University Press, ch 2.

Vohra, S. (in process) 'Review of impact assessments from a health perspective' (title to be confirmed – research being undertaken on behalf of the Department of Health).

Wanless, D. (2002) *Securing our future health: Taking a long-term view, Final report*, London: HM Treasury.

Wanless, D. (2004) *Securing good health for the whole population, Final report*, London: Department of Health.

Wanless, D., Appleby, J., Harrison, A. and Patel, D. (2007) *Our future health secured? A review of NHS funding and performance*, London: King's Fund.

Webster, C. (1992) 'Public health in decline', *Health Matters*, 11: 10-11.

Webster, C. (2002) *The National Health Service: A political history*, Oxford: Oxford University Press.

Which? (2005) *Choice: Health*, London: *Which?*.

WHO (World Health Organization) (1948) *Official Records of the WHO*, no 2, p 100.

WHO (1978) *Report on the International Conference on Primary Care, Alma Ata*, Geneva: WHO.

WHO (1981) *Global strategy for 'Health for All by the Year 2000'*, Geneva: WHO.

WHO (1986) *Ottawa Charter for Health Promotion*, Geneva: WHO.

WHO (2002) *The World Health Report 2002: Reducing risks, promoting healthy life*, Geneva: WHO.

WHO (2003) *Framework Convention on Tobacco Control*, Geneva: WHO (www.who.int/tobacco/framework/WHO_FCTC_english.pdf).

WHO (2006) *Climate change and human health – risks and responses: Summary*, Geneva: WHO (www.who.int/globalchange/climate/summary/en/).

WHO (2008a) *Closing the gap in a generation: Health equity through action on the social determinants of health*, Commission on Social Determinants of Health, Geneva: WHO.

WHO (2008b) *Guidelines for implementation of Article 5.3 of the WHO Framework Convention on Tobacco Control on the protection of public health policies with respect to tobacco control from commercial and other vested interests of the tobacco industry*, Geneva: WHO (www.who.int/fctc/guidelines/article_5_3.pdf).

WHO (2008c) *Primary health care now more than ever*, Geneva: WHO.

WHO (2008d) *The Tallinn Charter: Health systems for health and wealth*, WHO European Ministerial Conference on 'Health systems: health systems, health and wealth', Tallinn, Estonia, 25-27 June, Copenhagen: WHO.

Wilkinson, D., Ferguson, M., Bowyer, C., Brown, J., Ladefogod, A., Monkhouse, C. et al (2004) *Sustainable development in the European Commission's integrated impact assessments for 2003*, London: Institute for European Environmental Policy.

Wilkinson, E. (2006) 'The UK's public health paradox', *The Lancet* 368(3538), 831-2.

Wilkinson, R. and Pickett, K. (2009) *The spirit level: Why more equal societies almost always do better*, London: Allen Lane.

Williams, S.J., Calnan, M. and Dolan, A. (2007) 'Explaining inequalities in health: theoretical, conceptual and methodological agendas', in E. Dowler and N. Spencer (eds) *Challenging health inequalities: From Acheson to 'Choosing Health'*, Bristol: The Policy Press.

Wills, J. and Woodhead, D. (2004) '"The glue that binds …": articulating values in multi-disciplinary public health', *Critical Public Health*, 14(1), 7-15.

Winslow. C.E.A. (1920) 'The untilled fields of public health', *Science* 51(1306), 23-33.

Wismar, M., Lahtinen, E., Stahl, T., Ollila, E. and Leppo, K. (2006) 'Introduction', in T. Stohl, M. Wismar, E. Ollila, E. Lahtinen and K. Leppo (eds) *Health in All Policies: Prospects and potential*, Helsinki: Ministry of Social Affairs and Health Finland and European Observatory on Health Systems and Policies.

Wright, J. (2007) 'Developing the public health workforce', in S. Griffiths and D.J. Hunter (eds) *New perspectives in public health* (2nd edn), Oxford: Radcliffe Publishing.

Index